T0220558

SURVIVING SPACE

SURVIVING SPACE
Papers on Infant Observation

ESSAYS ON THE CENTENARY OF
Esther Bick

Edited by
Andrew Briggs

Foreword by
Donald Meltzer

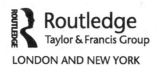

Routledge
Taylor & Francis Group

LONDON AND NEW YORK

Chapter 1 (pp. 27–36), "Child Analysis Today", Chapter 2 (pp. 37–54), "Notes on Infant Observation in Psycho-Analytic Training", and Chapter 3 (pp. 55–59), "The Experience of the Skin in Early Object Relations", by Esther Bick reproduced by permission from *Collected Papers of Martha Harris and Esther Bick,* ed. M. Harris Williams (Strathtay, Perthshire: Clunie Press, 1987).

Chapter 4 (pp. 60–71), "Further Considerations on the Function of the Skin in Early Object Relations", by Esther Bick reproduced by permission from *British Journal of Psychotherapy*, 2 (No. 4, 1986): 292–299.

Extracts on pp. 164–167 reprinted by permission from F. Donati, "Madness and Morale: A Chronic Psychiatric Ward", in R. D. Hinshelwood & W. Skogstad (Eds.), *Observing Organisations* (London: Routledge, 2000).

First published 2002 by Karnac Books Ltd.

Published 2019 by Routledge
2 Park Square, Milton Park, Abingdon, Oxon OX14 4RN
52 Vanderbilt Avenue, New York, NY 10017, USA

Routledge is an imprint of the Taylor & Francis Group, an informa business

British Library Cataloguing in Publication Data
A C.I.P. for this book is available from the British Library

ISBN 9781855752924 (pbk)

Edited, designed, and produced by Communication Crafts

CONTENTS

v

II
Pushing at the boundaries

SERIES EDITORS' PREFACE

Since it was founded in 1920, the Tavistock Clinic has developed a wide range of therapeutic approaches to mental health which have been strongly influenced by the ideas of psychoanalysis. It has also adopted systemic family therapy as a theoretical model and a clinical approach to family problems. The Clinic is now the largest training institution in Britain for mental health, providing postgraduate and qualifying courses in social work, psychology, psychiatry, and child, adolescent, and adult psychotherapy, as well as in nursing and primary care. It trains about 1,400 students each year in over 45 courses.

The Clinic's philosophy aims at promoting therapeutic methods in mental health. Its work is founded on the clinical expertise that is also the basis of its consultancy and research activities. The aim of this Series is to make available to the reading public the clinical, theoretical, and research work that is most influential at the Tavistock Clinic. The Series sets out new approaches in the understanding and treatment of psychological disturbance in children, adolescents, and adults, both as individuals and in families.

Surviving Space traces the origins of infant observation and describes the way in which it has developed and been applied. In so doing, the book combines some of the most established and the most original aspects of the clinical method, training, and research that lie at the heart of the Tavistock approach.

In celebration of the centenary of her birth, the four pioneering papers of Mrs Esther Bick are reprinted here, together with a number of essays that draw on and elaborate the insights implicit and explicit in her ideas. The theoretical innovativeness of her original papers is illuminated in a number of lively discussions that focus, in particular, on the difficulties of engaging with infants and young children whose very early development has been seriously impaired to the point where the self's survival is in question.

Further essays extend the central discoveries beyond the clinical setting to broader areas—legal, cultural, research, and organizational—in each case stressing the impact of more primitive emotional states, the understanding of which underlies Mrs Bick's unique contribution both within the psychoanalytic community and far beyond.

Nicholas Temple and Margot Waddell
Series Editors

ACKNOWLEDGEMENTS

The idea of putting together a festschrift for Mrs Bick was born from discussions I had with R. D. Hinshelwood in the middle of 2001. We both recognized the need to mark the centenary of such a remarkable woman, who has made such an impact in the psychoanalytic world. This led on to discussions with Karl Figlio and Margaret Rustin, through which we maintained that the focus should be on Mrs Bick's contribution to child psychotherapy. Child psychotherapists and others were approached to write short papers on what I knew of their special experience or expertise with her ideas. The preliminary discussions and editing the work of these distinguished writers have been a privilege. Through them I now know a great deal more about Mrs Bick, her work, and its contemporary applications than I did when I first asked them to contribute. However, as I have discovered, the editor's job has a share of difficult tasks too. Of these, I found the maintenance of the length of each contribution the most difficult. This required negotiations with an author that would end with some very rich and still valuable material on the cutting-room floor. I thank the authors for their generosity in making what was a painful task for us that much easier. The photographs reproduced in this book were kindly supplied by Mary Boston (p. xxii) and Judith Elkan (p. xxiv).

While I take full responsibility for this production, others deserve great thanks as their support has helped it come into being. Oliver Rathbone, at Karnac, played an early role with his keen interest in this project, as did Leena Häkkinen. Margot Waddell was very generous and strong with her support of the project and, with Nick Temple, worked behind the scenes as the general editors for the Series. Numerous people asked me how work was progressing, and some have been generous with their time and thoughts. Without making a distinction, among them I would like to mention Mary Boston, Sophie Boswell, Beta Copley, Judith Elkan, Athol Hughes, Betty Joseph, Trudy Klauber, Ros Lazar, Donald Meltzer, Marja Schulman, Roger Willoughby, and Isca Wittenberg. However, special mention is for my wife, Marigemma Rocco-Briggs, who helped me create enough space in our lives to think more clearly about the project. For this, I am enormously grateful.

ABOUT THE CONTRIBUTORS

Anne Alvarez is a Consultant Child and Adolescent Psychotherapist and recently retired from her position as Co-Convener of the Autism Service, Child and Family Department, Tavistock Clinic. She lectures for the M.A. and Doctoral programmes of the Tavistock/University of East London courses in Psychoanalytic Psychotherapy and in Observational Studies. She is author of *Live Company: Psychotherapy with Autistic, Borderline, Deprived and Abused Children* (1992) and has edited, with Susan Reid, *Autism and Personality: Findings from the Tavistock Autism Workshop* (1999).

Andrew Briggs is a Consultant Child Psychotherapist in the London Borough of Havering and Fellow of the Centre for Psychoanalytic Studies at the University of Essex. He has a particular interest in infant observation and has been a seminar leader for students from disciplines other than child psychotherapy. He is currently researching the historical development of child psychotherapy in the NHS.

Stephen Briggs is Senior Clinical Lecturer, Vice Dean of Post Graduate Studies and Head of Social Work in the Adolescent Department of the Tavistock Clinic. He is author of *Growth and Risk in Infancy* (1997) and of *Working with Adolescents: A Contemporary Psychodynamic Approach* (2002).

Jan Dollery graduated from Goldsmith's college in 1975, since when she has taught mainly in the field of special education. In 1985 she was appointed as an advisory/support teacher for Traveller children. In February 2001 she presented a paper, "The Emotional Development of Children within the Traveller Community and the Implications for Their Formal Education", at an International Symposium in Naples. She is currently a student on a regional psychoanalytical observational course associated with the Tavistock Clinic.

R. D. Hinshelwood is a Member of the British Psychoanalytical Society and Fellow of the Royal College of Psychiatrists. He is Professor in the Centre for Psychoanalytical Studies, University of Essex; previously Clinical Director, The Cassel Hospital; founder of the *British Journal of Psychotherapy*; and Past-Chair, The Association of Therapeutic Communities. He is the author of several books, including *A Dictionary of Kleinian Thought* (1991), *Clinical Klein* (1993), *Therapy or Coercion* (1997), and *Thinking about Institutions* (2001). He is co-editor of *Observing Organisations* (2000), with Wilhelm Skogstad, and of *Organisations, Anxiety and Defence* (2001), with Marco Chiesa.

Judith Jackson is a Child Psychotherapist and Child and Adult Psychoanalyst. She is a Member of the British Psychoanalytical Society. She is Organising Tutor for the Tavistock-linked Observational Studies programme at the Lincoln Centre, where she is also Director of Studies for the Adult Psychotherapy training. She has taught in Italy and South Africa and now teaches Infant Observation at the Tavistock Clinic and the British Institute of Psychoanalysis. She has published in the *Journal of Child Psychotherapy* and the *Journal of Infant Observation*. She is in private practice with children and adults.

Jeanne Magagna trained as a Child, Adult, and Family psychotherapist at the Tavistock Clinic. She is Head of Psychotherapy

Services at Great Ormond Street Hospital in London and is the Joint Coordinator of the Centro Studi Martha Harris Child Psychotherapy Training in Florence, Italy. She specializes in work with eating-disordered children and also works with the Ellernmede Centre for Eating Disorders in London.

Eleanor Nowers is a Psychoanalyst in private practice. She is an Associate Member of the British Psychoanalytical Society.

Maria Rhode is a Consultant Child and Adolescent Psychotherapist at the Tavistock Clinic in London, where she is a tutor on the Child Psychotherapy training. She has a particular interest in autism, language development, and infant observation and has contributed papers and book chapters on these topics. She is co-editor, with Margaret Rustin and Alex and Hélène Dubinsky, of *Psychotic States in Children* (1997) and is presently co-editing, with Trudy Klauber, a book on Asperger's Syndrome.

Michael Rustin is Professor of Sociology at the University of East London and a Visiting Professor at the Tavistock Clinic. He is author of *The Good Society and the Inner World* (1991) and *Reason and Unreason: Psychoanalysis, Science and Politics* (2001); co-author, with Margaret Rustin, of *Narratives of Love and Loss* (1989/2001) and *Mirror to Nature* (2002); and a co-editor of *Closely Observed Infants* (1987).

Joan Symington is a Child Psychiatrist and Psychoanalyst. She was Consultant Child Psychiatrist at the Royal Free Hospital for ten years. Having trained at the British Psychoanalytical Society, she now works in Sydney and is a Training Analyst of the Australian Psychoanalytical Society. She has published articles on infant observation and psychoanalysis. She is co-author, with her husband Neville, of *The Clinical Thinking of Wilfred Bion* 1996) and editor of the Sydney Klein Festschrift, *Imprisoned Pain and Its Transformation* (2000).

Biddy Youell is a Consultant Child and Adolescent Psychotherapist in the Child and Family Department of the Tavistock Clinic and at the Monroe Young Family Centre. She is Organizing Tutor of the Tavistock/University of East London MA programme, "Emotional Factors in Learning and Teaching", and has a particular interest in the application of psychoanalytic ideas in non-clinical settings.

FOREWORD

Donald Meltzer

A t the time of her death, Mrs Bick was hardly known except to her pupils, a number of whom have contributed to this volume. The reasons for this relative anonymity are to be sought in her modesty, which, as with Roger Money-Kyrle, led her to avoid public display. She did not, and could not, make public appearances, nor write books and papers. In fact, the few pregnant papers that have survived were produced in a kind of supervision/dictation to Martha Harris. But as a teacher she was outstanding, passionate, turbulent, and inspiring.

Although she had been well trained as a psychologist in scientific method, she had very little use for evidence and linear, logical thought or causality. Her thought was unequivocally intuitive, lateral, and poetic. Consequently the student never really could grasp her method or follow her thinking. Like Bion, her method of observation was so introspective that her conclusions appeared as groundless, hanging in mid-air by threads of conviction. Her demeanour forbade challenging and argument as the listener somehow osmosed the conviction. Nothing was invented, but her keenness of observation made sparkling discoveries of psychic reality and its phenomena. In retrospect, these discoveries may seem obvious, even banal, like the functions of the skin, or fanciful, like the types of second-skin formation. Never a theoretician, she was, rather, a naturalist, observing and reporting phenomena and enabling others to see, to receive the vibrations, hear the music, and smell the scent of love and hate in its primitive forms.

These qualities placed her firmly beside Melanie Klein and the best in Freud and Bion. It is not, therefore, so surprising that along with this volume of papers, the gradual growth of infant observation carried forth by her students has begun to produce a blossoming literature in France (Michel Haag), in Barcelona (the group around Berman), and in Portugal and Sweden (Johan Norman's group).

Esther Bick was that rare creature: an inspiring teacher.

THE LIFE AND WORK OF ESTHER BICK

Esther Bick was born Esteza Lifsza Wander, on 4 July 1902, to an impoverished orthodox Jewish family living near the fortress town of Przemyśl, in Galicia, on the Ukrainian border of the Austro-Hungarian Empire. She died on 20 July 1983 in a nursing home in Gants Hill, Essex. She was a founder of child psychotherapy, and through her teaching at the Tavistock Clinic in the postwar years she played an important role in establishing child psychotherapy as a profession (A. Briggs, forthcoming).

In her obituary for Esther Bick, Martha Harris (1983) paid tribute to her courage, perseverance, and intelligence, saying that she left "her profession and the world a richer place". She referred to Esther Bick's introduction of infant observation to the core of the child psychotherapist's training as "a stroke of genius" and to her papers on this and child analysis as seminal and remaining so. Having spoken to some of Esther Bick's students and colleagues, I think we need to add "determined" and "pioneering" to these qualities and, furthermore, to acknowledge that her seminal influence continues not only through her writings, but also through the lasting impact of her personality on those she supervised and taught.

Now, in Esther Bick's centenary year and looking back over the past nineteen years since Martha Harris wrote her obituary, it is clear that her ideas have remained at the cutting edge of our thinking and are still today, as during her lifetime, enabling child psychotherapists to develop new insights and understanding. During the fifty-three years of the profession, the work of the child psychotherapist has become increasingly more difficult and varied, with new patient populations and developments in the work setting presenting opportunities for fresh avenues in our thinking, as the chapters in this festschrift reflect.   Before we turn in part I to Bick's ideas and then in part II to our contributors' development of them, I shall give a brief overview of her life, hoping to convey something of her qualities as a person, a seminar leader, and a supervisor.

Courage, determination, perseverance, and intelligence

In 1983, in the very last year of her life, Esther Bick was interviewed by Jeanne Magagna and Hélène Dubinsky, two of her students, and she described to them some of the formative experiences of her early life. At the age of 7 years, she was sent from Przemyśl to assist her aunt in Prague, who had just had a baby. For three years she helped her aunt to raise the baby, and then she returned home. At around the age of 15 or 16 she applied for work as a nursery teacher, and she persuaded the hiring agency that she was suitable for work with children because of her experiences at home. On the first morning at the nursery, finding that she could not control two of the children, she was on the point of resigning. She decided instead, however, to learn how to do the work by spending the afternoons observing the teacher who ran the afternoon session. One of her purposes in doing nursery work had been to earn money to fulfil her passion of going to Israel. Sadly, this plan was shelved because her father died during this period and, as the eldest child, she had to help bring up her siblings. She later said: "Doing this and working at the nursery made me decide to become a child psychologist" (Magagna & Dubinsky, 1983).

The problem she faced in having made this decision to become a psychologist was her lack of consistent schooling, which put her at considerable disadvantage when thinking about university entrance. However, obviously determined, not only did she study, on her own and in one year, all the subjects for the Baccalaureate that students at school took seven years to cover, but she passed the examinations in all of them except mathematics. She later re-sat this examination successfully, having been prepared for it by a young university student.[1] Initially she had planned to go to Switzerland to study with Jean Piaget, but she was turned down because that country was not accepting foreigners. Instead, she went to Vienna to study under Charlotte Bühler, who was then researching infant development through detailed study of individual babies from birth. Although—as Bick recalled in later life—she had been uncomfortable with the behavioural approach of the research, in 1936 she completed her Ph.D. thesis, entitled "Observations of the Two and a Half Year Old". She expressed her discomfort with this approach during an interview with Jeanne Magagna, saying that it was "really behaviouristic . . . just terrible". She had to use a stopwatch to study and count the children's social responses to each other. This experience, she said, led to her wanting to study "the ordinary life of babies" in their own "family environment". [2] She expressed similar sentiments in the interview with Magagna and Dubinsky (1983):

> I was given two two and a half year old children to observe. I was to count the times child X responded to child Y, and the times child Y responded to child X. I faithfully recorded and counted all the responses, but I was determined I would someday study what I observed which couldn't be quantified.

When she first went to study in Vienna, she needed to find unofficial work because her university fees, as a foreigner, were high, and her family were unable to assist her financially. Early on, she lived with a family and looked after their young child. She left

---

[1] A. Gardziel (2002) has researched Esther Bick's school experiences in Przemysl.

[2] Jeanne Magagna, personal communication.

this to work, from 1930 to 1936, in a children's home run by
Marianne Prager, who was to become a life-long friend. Within this
period, in 1934, she also became an assistant to Charlotte Bühler.
As if these duties were not enough while studying at university,
she also trained as a teacher. On leaving university, she used this
qualification to work with 7-year-olds. It was at this time that she
married a medical student, Phillip Bick. [3]

The German invasion of Vienna in March 1938 was the beginning of several especially precarious moments in the life of Esther
Bick. The Gestapo came for her husband one evening; they said
they would remain outside the house until he returned, but she
escaped to another part of the city to find him. In the interview
with Magagna and Dubinsky (1983), Esther Bick said that she and
her husband crossed into Switzerland without their guide, who
had been captured, and they found safety with the Jewish refugee
organization there. What happened to Mr Bick after this is not
clear. [4]

While exactly how the marriage ended remains uncertain, it is
clear that Esther Bick arrived in England without her husband. She
had not, as a foreigner, been allowed to work in Switzerland, and
she was sent by the refugee camp to stay in London with Eva
Hauser, the sister of one of the camp's administrators, who was to
become another of her few close friends in England. Bick joined the
Society of British University Women and, in July 1939, took up
their offer of a two-week holiday in Suffolk on the country estate of
Miss Violet Oates, whose famously selfless brother had walked out
into the Antarctic snow. She struck up a friendship with Violet
Oates—who, she said, was more impressive than her brother could
have been—and she stayed with her until Christmas of that year.

From Suffolk she went to Manchester, where Marianne Prager
was working in a hostel for refugee boys. Again she first worked
looking after a child, but soon she was teaching in a wartime day
nursery in Salford. Here she acquired a reputation for thinking
about what children might be experiencing and for trying to make
the staff aware that their own practices had profound effects on the

---

[3] In the public domain nothing else is known of Mr Bick.
[4] There are many areas of Mrs Bick's life that remain unclear, her life in
Austria and Switzerland being particularly so.

children. She also noticed that the children's agitation and disturbance was quieted when she gave each child pebbles and an empty
can into which to put them (see chapter 6). The reason behind this
activity seems so obvious now, but at that time it represented a real
discovery about containment. During this period she went into
analysis with Michael Balint, who had arrived from Budapest in
1939. Between 1942 and 1945 she worked one day a week in a child
guidance clinic in Leeds. This work introduced her to the writings
on child analysis of both Anna Freud and Melanie Klein.

At the end of the war, Bick returned to London. Balint had also
moved there, and she continued her analysis with him. She took a
job at Ealing child guidance clinic, where she particularly enjoyed
her first case—a 9-year-old boy whom she saw with his grandmother. In 1947 Balint encouraged her to apply to train at the
Institute of Psychoanalysis, and she was accepted. Her supervisors
there were James Strachey and Melanie Klein. Klein supervised
her second adult and first child cases, and Bick was very impressed by her. With Balint's agreement, she terminated her analysis with him and started with Klein. One of her interviewers for
the Institute had been Dr John Bowlby, and Esther Bick later recalled that

> A few weeks later he 'phoned me asking if I'd like to work as a
> child psychotherapist at the Tavistock Clinic. . . . I began doing
> psychotherapy with children at the Tavistock. By the autumn I
> had begun a small seminar to discuss children. Dr Bowlby was
> part of that group. [Magagna & Dubinsky, 1983]

Bick's unambiguously Kleinian position and the ethology of
Bowlby would suggest an unusual combination from the start. In
1948, they jointly started the first child psychotherapy training at
the Tavistock, and infant observation was given central place. [5] By
1960 they had parted company as course directors. This might not
have been inevitable, had they been able to agree to differ over
their own positions on attachment and separation. However, the
potential for such a working relationship seems to have been rather
stretched by matters other than the epistemological and clinical.
Martha Harris, in her obituary, also mentioned that Esther Bick

---

[5] Mary Boston, personal communication.

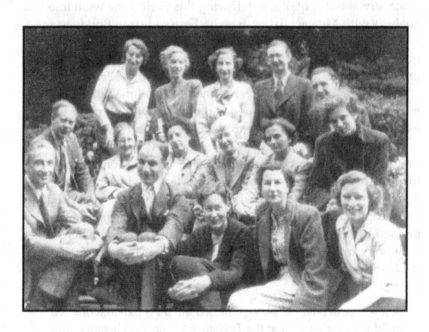

Photograph taken in 1949 or 1950 by James Robertson in the garden of the Tavistock Clinic's original site in Beaumont Street, West London. Esther Bick is third from the left in the middle row, John Bowlby is on the far left of the same row.

(From left to right) Front row: Dugmore Hunter; Paul Davies; Mary Boston; Barbara Michaels; Martha Harris. *Middle row*: John Bowlby; Noel Hunnybun; Esther Bick; Constance Simmins; Yana Popper; Dina Rosenbluth. *Back row*: Mrs Ursula Bowlby; Doris Wills; Elizabeth Brown; Robert Todd; Julian Katz.

was not known for her diplomatic skills, and this led to Bowlby telling her that "he would not be asking her to take responsibility for another intake of students" (Harris, 1983). Donald Meltzer, who was a supervisee and later a colleague of Bick, is certain that her part in the difficulties with Bowlby was due to the dogmatic and uncompromising stance she took about the rightness and clarity of her own views.[6] To some extent her students also saw this quality in her. Although not party to the exact nature of their course leaders' differences, some of the tension was experienced as "something going on" by the students who trained during those years. [7] Others mention that the views taken on cases by Bowlby and Bick were rather obviously different. It was clear that Bowlby's analysis and categorization of material and Bick's view of striving to think about what could be seen in it and what that meant in terms of the inner world were starkly at variance with each other.

Far more research about Esther Bick's life and work is obviously needed, but what remains clear so far is her courage, perseverance, and determination to see things through. An early life spent looking after children led first to teaching, then to research, and finally to analysing them. Having completed her doctorate with Charlotte Bühler, she was determined to study something she had seen about children, and the process of observing them, but which could not be quantified. By the time she became a supervisor or seminar leader, this study was something like a determined quest each time she was presented with clinical material.

Seminar leader, supervisor, and pioneer

No longer responsible after 1960 for the running of Tavistock training, Esther Bick continued as seminar leader and also supervised students training at the Tavistock and at the Institute of Psychoanalysis. Although many recognized more than a hint of their fear when with her, most were in awe of her capacity for clear and

---

[6] Dr Meltzer, personal communication.
[7] Judith Elkan, personal communication.

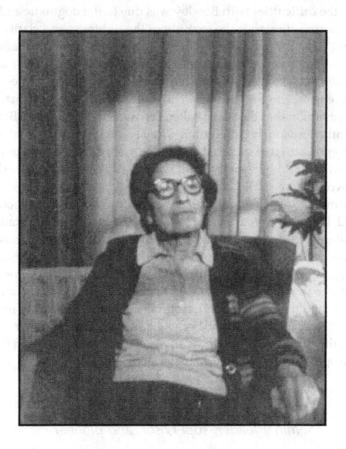

Esther Bick [1902–1983]

highly original thinking. This awe was not necessarily amplified by their knowing little about her as a person. She was very private, and so much of what was then known about her came through noticing aspects of her that she did not keep quiet, such as her exceptional physical energy. It has been said that in her late seventies she was still easily able to climb the stairs to her fourth-floor flat in North London. All experienced her warmth as she welcomed them to seminar groups or supervisions with freshly made apple strudel.

The energy and vitality she exuded when focusing upon her students' material was, as most said, inspirational. Insisting on detailed verbatim written observations—from newly qualified or experienced child psychotherapists or colleagues alike—she would ask questions, searching to find what else happened in particular scenarios. In this volume, the chapters by Jeanne Magagna (chapter 5) and Joan Symington (chapter 6) bring to life the experience of taking material to her and watching her follow it by asking for more detail before making brilliantly insightful comments. What is so immediately obvious from these chapters, and from the accounts given to me by some of her other students, is Bick's unique gift of being in touch with the baby and his earliest moments of life.[8] Through this, as her papers on the experience of the skin so graphically convey (1968, 1986), she became in touch with the newborn's struggle for survival. As one of her students put it: "I don't know that anybody has been so in touch with the early survival mechanisms of the infant."[9]

This gift of empathy with the newborn was something that, through her teaching, she shared with her students. For this they forgave her her dogmatic approach to their presentations and thinking, as through it they learnt more about their material and her method for understanding it. Esther Bick was very convinced of her own views, and in her seminars students were not encouraged to have their own associations to the material presented. Indeed, those who tried did not meet with a good reception by her.

---

[8] Throughout, for simplicity, in general discussions masculine pronouns have been used for the infant or young child.

[9] Isca Wittenberg, personal communication.

The presentations had to come up to her very exacting standards. She would often take written notes as the presenter read his or her written verbatim account of an observation, stopping the delivery to ask for more detail. Each new detail was thought about, and often more was asked for before the reader was allowed to proceed. Esther Bick would savour what she heard, visibly think about it, and give her opinion in very carefully chosen, often vivid, words that conveyed that she had gone right to the heart of the matter, before imparting exactly what she saw there. When she spoke, it was always clear and graphic. Judith Elkan, also as graphically, describes Esther Bick empathically moving towards an understanding of the infant in focus:

> As she delved into the world of the infant, it was as if she went underwater, and swum around in the world of the infant's mind and then surfaced and related what she had found there. She would sink into the depths, and then emerge and would be piecing together some of the information that she'd noted. When she told us what she had seen, it then gradually emerged to become clear for us students. [10]

Esther Bick's search for meaning was to have a seminal influence on her students and, through them, on the next generation of child psychotherapists whom they sensitively inducted into her method and thinking. Indeed, such was her passion for finding out about the experiences of the child that students who visited her in the last days of her life were surprised to be met by her questions about their work, upon which she was still able to make characteristically insightful comments.

There is much more that could be said about the life of this remarkable woman. In conveying some of her experiences and something about her contribution to child psychotherapy, I hope to have given a sense of her courage, her determination to study something that she had seen long before she arrived in England, and her perseverance with making sure she found a way of studying it once she settled here. That she brought these qualities to her clinical and teaching work is evident in the reflections of her students. They are also clear in her papers.

---

[10] Judith Elkan, personal communication.

A reluctant writer

Esther Bick's four well-known papers, reprinted here in part I, were all written in the twenty-year period between the early 1960s and the early 1980s. There is at least one, but possible three other papers, in the public domain written by her. The first of these, "Anxieties Underlying Phobia of Sexual Intercourse in a Woman", found in the archives of Clifford Scott, was recently published (Bick, 2001). [11] She read this paper to a Scientific Meeting of the British Psychoanalytical Society in June 1953, where she was elected a Full Member. There is a record of her previously having presented two other papers. One of these, "Notes on a Case of a Boy Treated on a Once a Week Basis", read in April 1948, followed her election as an Associate Member. In May 1948 she read "Psychoanalytic Work in Child Guidance". There is an archive record of both of these titles, but there is no evidence that they still exist. [12]

Considering a career of such importance and length, for us this is a sad paucity of publications. Esther Bick was known to have been extremely reluctant to write. In a discussion of her second paper on the function of the skin, published posthumously in 1986, Meltzer refers to this reluctance as depriving "us of a record of the scope of her observation and ideas" (1986a, p. 300). With this in mind, it needs to be emphasized that she is known to have disliked writing, and her papers were produced only after persuasion by two of the students closest to her, Martha Harris and Donald Meltzer.[13] Explanations for this dislike have tended to emphasize her intense self-criticism, which drove her to achieve perfection in all that she applied herself to.

This concept of perfection did not simply mean that she avoided writing because she could never be content that she had conveyed exactly what she had in mind; it was more that she was striving with herself to better understand what she had observed and thus had in mind. Meltzer (1974) certainly conveys this in remembering their preliminary discussions on what was later to be

---

[11] This paper was discovered by Roger Willoughby during his doctoral research. He published (Willoughby, 2001) a very interesting appraisal of this early paper in the same issue of the journal as that in which the paper appeared.

[12] Pearl King, Riccardo Steiner, and Jill Duncan, personal communications.

[13] Dr Meltzer, personal communication.

written about as adhesive identification. These started out as discussions on the identification processes of the patients she was describing. He recounts Bick describing her observation that certain of her patients had previously overcome severe states of anxiety through their idiosyncratic "secondary skin formations" or "substitute skin formations". Very focused on the sensual aspect of what she saw, she was left with a feeling that she was unable to conceptualize. She told Meltzer that "they are sticky, they stick" (Meltzer, 1974, p. 344) and "Oh. I don't know how to talk about it, they are just like that [sticking her hands together]. It is something different" (p. 336). Such was her determination that she persevered with her attempt to put into as satisfactory words as possible a feeling that she thought had a huge bearing on better understanding her patients. Meltzer remembers her struggling with the difficulty presented by the inadequacy of having to use words—which she said were "slippery" and did not adequately convey what she was observing—to describe what happens in the sensual domain inhabited by the infant.[14] I think this begins to explain why she was not comfortable with either the spoken or written word as a medium through which to convey experiences from clinical work. The extent to which this had a bearing on the quantity of her written output needs to be researched. However, it does begin to help us understand why she spoke and wrote in such a graphic way.

* * *

This brief description of the life and work of Esther Bick has been no more than a sketch. However, I hope I have managed to convey something of her spirit, a spirit that can also be seen in the growth of the things she was passionate about. Infant observation, child analysis, and psychotherapy have all flourished through the enterprise of the generations of workers who have benefited directly from her teaching. As the Introduction shows, her ideas continue to remain strong and are still being developed and elaborated, and her spirit adds to the strength of passion for those who use and develop them.

[14] Dr Meltzer, personal communication.

SURVIVING SPACE

Introduction

E sther Bick brought new thinking to psychoanalysis, and
to the psychoanalysis of children in particular. Her method
of discovery—infant observation—allowed her to swim in
the depths of the baby's experience and to emerge with unique
insights into the terrors facing any newborn and his desperate
attempts to create a psychic space in which to survive. She suc-
cinctly reported her findings in a series of innovative papers on the
experience and function of the skin in early object relations. Her
centenary provides an opportunity to take stock of her ideas and
their use today.

Esther Bick was undoubtedly an important figure in the British
Psychoanalytical Society, but she also had a colossal impact on the
origins and development of child psychotherapy, and the collection of essays in this book derives mainly from her influence on the
child psychotherapy training at the Tavistock Clinic. Her influence
has also spread to the teaching of other closely related disciplines.
Year after year, child psychotherapists are meeting increasing demands to run observation seminars for clinical psychologists,
counsellors, doctors, health visitors, school and college teachers,

and social workers. Infant observation has become a prime require-
ment of most psychodynamic training courses in Great Britain. It
has also become central to the development of mental health and
allied professionals in many countries, including those in Eastern
and Western Europe, India, and South America.

This book aims to provide a snapshot of particular kinds of
work, in both clinical and other settings, in which Esther Bick's
ideas are used or have been developed. It is particular for two
reasons: it focuses on the English-speaking world, and most of the
contributors are directly linked to child psychotherapy. However,
I hope that the end product will be valuable to all professionals
interested in Bick's ideas, regardless of nationality or specific
training. One can see that the contributors, although using different perspectives, are all grounded in Bick's thinking and develop
aspects of her papers in very original ways. Some of these can be
said to accentuate and explore ideas that she left implicit in her
writing. Others take her explicitly formed ideas a little further.
There are also chapters that show how her thinking can be used
outside the clinical and training settings in which she worked.
Overall, the authors each carry the spirit of Bick's pioneering en-
deavour, as they too push at the boundaries beyond what is familiar. Their chapters show that her ideas are dynamic and, without
compromising their original principles, are in a state of constant
evolution. There is no question that they are as important today as
they were when she first developed these ideas in the 1950s and
1960s.

We are pleased to be able to publish Esther Bick's four papers
with this collection, in part I. This allows some readers to discover
her ideas for the first time, others to reacquaint themselves with
them, and so to track their development in the other chapters, in
part II. For my part, I want briefly to discuss two ways in which
Bick's ideas were pioneering. First, infant observation, as a naturalistic means of generating understanding, helps us see the inner
world of the infant far more clearly than would otherwise have
been possible. Second, her focus on the infant's struggle for survival took our attention to an even earlier site of infant development than that visited by Melanie Klein. To say that this discussion
provides a backdrop to the following chapters would be misleading: Bick's ideas provide both background and foreground.

Infant observation: swimming in the depths

The universal appeal of Bick's method of infant observation is found in its versatility. In observing the earliest moments of a baby's life, students learn about the impact of emotional events on the development of the mind and about personal and social relationships specific to that infant. This experience leaves them with a way of thinking about the development of humans in general. Bick was not alone in developing this aspect of infant observation, as a not dissimilar approach was being used by Anna Freud and her colleagues.[1] What was, and remains, so important about Bick's method is her focus on the emotionality of the observer as a means by which to gain a clearer view of the infant. This was pioneering, and I want to suggest here that it was a great deal more so than Bick probably recognized.

Taken together, Bick's papers "Child Analysis Today" (1962 [chapter 1 herein]) and "Notes on Infant Observation in Psycho-Analytic Training" (1964 [chapter 2 herein]) become a full account of her method of observation, discovery, and thinking. In the latter she discusses how the trainee learns through observation to understand play and other nonverbal expressions of infantile experience more clearly, to recognize the impact of the baby on family dynamics, and to use these experiences to understand a child in treatment and make sense of the parents' account of the child's early life. However, to my mind, what also makes introducing infant observation to the training of child psychotherapists "a stroke of genius" (in the words of Martha Harris) is the way in which it enables the observer to develop a particular state of mind that allows for closer and more authentic observation. Prior to these two papers, issues around how to receive and think about material in an observation or clinical setting had not been discussed with such a detailed focus on method. It is my suggestion here that Bick, apparently unintentionally, built upon Freud's (1912e, 1923a [1922]) discussions about "evenly suspended attention", anticipated Bion's (1967) thoughts on memory and desire, and placed what Keats (1817) termed

---

[1] See, for example, Anna Freud's "Observations on Child Development" (1951), "Some Remarks on Infant Observation" (1953), and "The Contribution of Direct Child Observation to Psychoanalysis" (1957).

"negative capability" at the core of the observational and thus clinical method.[2] Furthermore, through the introduction of infant observation as a training method, Bick helped us begin to develop such a capability for ourselves.

The starting point for seeing Bick in this way is to suggest that infant observation is driven by what Keats had in mind when he said "Nothing ever becomes real till it is experienced" (1819). I think Keats's use of the words "real" and "experienced" should be placed beside his earlier definition of what he called negative capa- bility—"that is when a man is capable of being in uncertainties, Mysteries, doubts, without any irritable reaching after fact and reason" (1817). Hence, I would suggest, "real" means that which is experienced for itself, free from any preconception by the observer. This requires a very special gift for observation. One of Keats's biographers, Stephen Coote, argues that the term "negative" gains explanation from Keats's studying chemistry as a medical student. Here, negative implies "a sympathetic receptive intensity" (Coote, 1995, p. 115). Bick was very good at helping her students to become aware of their own preconceptions.   [3] In this she facilitated their development of this capacity for negative capability, because she saw preconceptions as getting in the way of a highly tuned capac- ity to observe, or experience, something for what it really is. The development of this capacity, I would suggest, is the *raison d'être* of Bick's observational method. The following is a very clear example of the imperative to have no preconceptions if one is to observe intensely:

> One may have to sit with children for a long time completely in
> the dark about what is going on, until suddenly something
> comes up from the depth that illuminates it. . . . [1962, p. 31
> herein]

This experience is like watching for a pattern to emerge, something one of her supervisees refers to as "waiting for something to

---

[2] Bion did not write about "negative capability" until 1970, in *Attention and Interpretation*. Although his ideas on this are evident in the chapter "Container and Contained", they are more developed in another chapter, "Prelude to or Substitute for Achievement".

[3] Dr Meltzer, personal communication.

emerge from the mist". [4] In waiting, without preconceptions, the observer's own depths become important:

> [This] imposes on the child analyst a greater dependence on his unconscious to provide him with clues to the meaning of the child's play and non-verbal communications. [1962, p. 31 herein]

That said, Bick recognized that an unquestioning dependence on clues from the unconscious was fraught with serious difficulties. These included internal "stresses" on the observer's capacity to see situations clearly. She describes the internal stresses the child psychotherapist is exposed to when waiting for something to come "up from the depth", through "the unique opportunity for intimate contact with primitive layers of the child's unconscious mind", which exposes us to "the constant problem of his unconscious identifications" (1962, p. 30 herein). Here she is examining how the intensity of the child's negative and positive transference in the therapeutic relationship arouses unconscious anxieties in the psychotherapist.

In her 1964 paper, Bick continues the discussion about training and the problem of stresses in observational and clinical work. She considers what "interferes with" the observer's capacity for free-floating attention and prevents him or her from observing the emotional needs of the mother and baby. This discussion, movingly illustrated by material from two observations (K and Charles), brings into focus not only the role of the observer but also that of the seminar group. The latter's role is to help the observer to "uncover some of the projections into him that are operating and which intensify his own internal conflicts" (1964, p. 39 herein). As in the 1962 paper, she recognizes the importance of being aware of projections as communicative. However, until they are seen as this, they have the potential to cloud the vision of the observer, possibly leading to a breaking of the role. The danger of such projections here is that they can obstruct the observer's ability to "resist being drawn into roles involving intense infantile transference and therefore countertransference" (p. 39 herein).

---

[4] Judith Elkan, personal communication.

The consequence of not resisting these roles is to be pulled into the family organization as, for example, a substitute mother for the baby, a sibling for an older child, or an emotional support for the mother. In this situation the observer has lost the capacity for "a sympathetic receptive intensity", as he or she has been unable to overcome the various stresses that observation brings. All the observational and training techniques having suffered a gradual or a rapid decline; the observer is left in a position where "his observations would then be as little objective as those of a father or mother student wanting to bring observations of their own" to the seminar (p. 39 herein). It is perhaps not surprising that Bick advocated that child analysts continued in personal analysis while they engaged in infant observation and for the duration of their clinical training.

Bick recognized the importance of being accurate in the use of language when describing observations. Her students report that she was very careful to use a word only if she was satisfied that it described, as exactly as possible, an observed action or thought about that action.[5] Her comment that "every word is loaded with a penumbra of implication" shows that she was very aware of how easily language clouds the observing lens that her method aimed to keep polished. When she discussed her students' observations, she would only proceed to a new observed action once clarity had been achieved on the previous one. This caution was undoubtedly a function of her wisdom, as she waited for discoveries to emerge in the sensual and other preverbal domains inhabited by the baby. In this way she extended the frontier, understanding linguistically what had been observed in these depths.

This caution and precision about language extended to her thinking about infant observation as a research method. Again, the idea of "negative capability" can speculatively be written into Bick's thoughts. This is especially so when one considers her comment that the researcher's aim is to "collect facts free from interpretation". This is obviously linked to her discussion of internal stresses. How these impede the researcher's thinking can be picked up in seminar groups through examining the language used to convey what is observed. With this focus on language she is clearly

---

[5] Judith Elkan, Isca Wittenberg, Dr Meltzer, personal communications.

recognizing that observing and thinking are "inseparable." Hence the development of meaning from what is initially observed needs to rely on "consecutive observations for confirmation" (1964, p. 51 herein). Only then can the patterns that emerge be termed hypotheses.

In both these papers there are other important ideas that are being developed by child psychotherapists and others today. However, one idea discussed in the 1962 paper, and often found in no small measure in current practice, is the tension between internal and external stresses, especially those brought about by the analyst's difficult position of being responsible both to the child and to the parents. The task here is to keep these two aspects in mind and to arrive at an appropriate balance between what is in the therapeutic interests of the child and what can be done to help alleviate any anxieties that may arise for the parents whose child is in treatment. In a passage that many will recognize as a succinct guide for working as a child psychotherapist, Bick recognizes that the importance of being clear about one's responsibility towards the child one is working with "may clash" with what others may want of us (1962, p. 29 herein).

There is much conceptual and practical thinking to be done if we are to develop further the insights that Bick had into the problem of achieving "negative capability"; my own thoughts on this are very much in their infancy. However, these two papers remind us of the dangers in thinking that we have solved mysteries when we have not first struggled with the various stresses inevitably involved in doing so.

The experience and function of the skin: surviving space

There can be little doubt that the two papers on the experience and function of the skin in early object relations (1968 [chapter 3 herein], 1986 [chapter 4 herein]) give us a new understanding of attachment, identity, separation, and loss. Bick achieved this by breaking fresh ground in two areas. First, she focused her attention on an earlier stage of preverbal development than had been exam-

ined in the works of Melanie Klein. It is clear that Bick had a
different understanding of the early moments of life and saw the
infant's ego developing later than Klein had done. The second area
takes us nearer to the pioneering developments that were taking
place in Bick's own clinical work and in her supervision of others.
This was her exploration of a site where communication and meaning are sensual, bodily, and reliant upon the various uses to which
the infant might put his sensory organs.

In her "Notes on Some Schizoid Mechanisms", Klein (1946) saw
the infant as having an ego at birth that can distinguish between
itself and its object. The infant therefore has some concept of himself and the object being separate. The recognition of such boundaries, with firmness and stability, allows for the capacity to introject
and project to become established. This is a crucial moment in the
ego's development, and crucial for the infant's sense of identity. By
the time she wrote this paper, Klein had moved away from the
classical idea, derived from Freud, that the ego has the task of
discharging instinctual tensions, mainly the death instinct. Rather,
she saw the ego as having experiences, and these were largely
brought about by phantasies and anxieties surrounding its complex relationship with its object.

In this paper Klein also saw the early ego oscillating between
states of integration and disintegration. She described the latter
as "a falling to bits" (1946, p. 4). This disintegration comes about
because the ego begins to recognize its existence as separate from
its object. Disintegration is understood as part of an attempt to
survive painful anxieties that are associated with this experience
and to defend against an overwhelming fear of annihilation. I think
that this is what she meant when she wrote that in the early moments of the ego, anxiety is "a fear of annihilation (death) and takes
the form of a fear of persecution . . . experienced as an uncontrollable overpowering object . . . the anxiety of being destroyed from
within" (pp. 4–5).

Klein therefore described the fear of disintegration as a primary
experience of the infant. She argued that the shifting states of integration and disintegration are connected with the appearance and
disappearance of the external good object. The loss of the internal
good object gives rise to extreme frustration, which is only eased
by the reappearance of the external good object for a resumption of

healthy introjection. Klein discussed the first introjection—that of the good and loved object—as creating an internal good object that becomes the core around which the early ego integrates: "The first internal object acts as a focal point in the ego. It counteracts the process of splitting and dispersal, makes for cohesiveness and integration, and is instrumental in building up the ego" (1946, p. 6). These persecutory fears have a deleterious effect on the infant's development if they become too strong, for if "the infant cannot work through the paranoid-schizoid position, the working through of the depressive position is in turn impeded" (p. 2).

Klein goes on to show the intricate details of the projections and introjections engaged in by the infant in the process of sustaining the ego and a sense of identity and in protecting himself from the fear of annihilation. In this paper Klein gives a comprehensive view of the struggle for survival that the very young infant is involved in. However, she does not address how an ego in pieces can perform these functions. For Bick, the "being in pieces" is a state for all infants until they are able to bind the parts of themselves together through contact with their object. Klein's paper had drawn attention to the early moments of the ego's existence. Bick's focused on even earlier moments, ones at the very beginning of *ex utero* life. In so doing she was able to draw attention to the infant's struggle to develop an ego and a sense of identity.

Bick's observations of babies led her to think about a situation prior to early ego formation. Unlike Klein, she did not believe that at birth the infant has an ego able to differentiate between itself and its object. Indeed, Bick saw the infant's earliest task as keeping his personality together, because inside him his most primitive parts were being experienced as having nothing to hold them together. This is what she is saying in the following often-quoted passage:

> in its most primitive form the parts of the personality are felt to have no binding force amongst themselves and must therefore be held together in a way that is experienced by them passively, by the skin functioning as a boundary. [1968, p. 55 herein]

With this statement Bick is suggesting not only a stage of development prior to the earliest one discussed by Klein, but a different reason for the sense of disintegration. Klein had argued that the falling to bits comes in the ebb and flow of the early ego's relationship with its internal and external objects. Bick identified an earlier stage of falling to bits, which is prior to the existence of an ego with the necessary boundary that allows for a sense of disintegration to occur, through splitting and projection. As she says,

> The stage of primal splitting and idealization of the self and object can . . . be seen to rest on this earlier process of containment of self and object by their respective "skins". [1968, p. 56 herein]

In this stage of development the baby's own skin, felt both from within itself and through its boundary with its mother's skin, is experienced as being able to hold together its personality. Hence, Bick was arguing that the first object is experienced by the baby as preventing disintegration. This is a passive experience. The object is only experienced from outside the self, and it is an experience that is not strived for by the infant. When this boundary has been successfully achieved, the function of the ego is to struggle for the capacity to introject.

> this internal function of containing the parts of the self is dependent initially on the introjection of an external object experienced as capable of fulfilling this function. . . . Until the containing functions have been introjected, the concept of a space within the self cannot arise. Introjection, i.e. construction of an object in an internal space, is therefore impaired. [1968, p. 56 herein]

The object needed here is the nipple in his mouth. As the achievement of this is dependent upon the mother's assistance, this is an active experience of acquisition. The concept of a space inside that holds the parts that make up his "self" is developed through sensing the mouth, a hole in the boundary of the skin, being closed with the arrival of the nipple. This space inside is thus felt as one into which the object can be introjected. Because the skin is a receptor organ, this introjection is sensual. Thus the baby identifies with the internal object because it becomes identified with his skin. Communication and experience are felt as sensual.

Klein drew our attention to the fact that in the paranoid-schizoid and depressive positions the infant has an internal object at the core of the ego. In drawing our attention to severe difficulties in the development of a capacity to introject, Bick took us to a stage prior to this. The relationship of this earlier stage to the paranoid-schizoid and depressive positions is obviously an important question, the answer to which is not readily available in Bick's papers. There is not the space here to develop a discussion, but I suggest that the falling to bits of the unheld infant does not seem to be the same as the disintegration that Klein mentions as a feature of the paranoid-schizoid position. In this sense it is not a persecutory phenomenon that results from introjection and projection. It has more the quality of the falling to bits in mourning, which is a feature of the depressive position and results from object loss.

The idea of the infant having to hold himself together does suggest that something has been lost that would otherwise have done this holding. Here the sensual experience of the mother's skin may have been momentarily introjected, just as the tactile experience of her body has been lost. The various ways of keeping the self together, which act as substitute skins, may then be ways of dealing with a falling to bits brought about by an acute feeling of loss. This raises the problem of identity, which is far too complicated to discuss in what is no more than a brief introduction to Bick's papers. Hence, one must conclude that when there is a capacity to introject, project, and lodge an internal object in the ego, identity can develop. When, as in secondary skin formation, this capacity is not developed, then neither is identity.

In her 1946 paper, Klein did not appear to recognize the difficulty of being able to introject and project in a disintegrated state. Bick takes this up in the concept of a failure during the passive stage of developing a skin. Without the experience of the mother's skin through the nipple in mouth, the infant desperately searches for a substitute. Bick describes this as follows:

> The need for a containing object would seem, in the infantile unintegrated state, to produce a frantic search for an object—a light, a voice, a smell, or other sensual object—which can hold the attention and thereby be experienced, momentarily at least, as holding the parts of the personality together. [1968, p. 56 herein]

Bick's thoughts on this kind of holding together, or containment, appear similar to Klein's view that, without a firm ego, the function and process of introjection and projection are severely impaired. However, she was also aware that an internal object was not achieved by all infants, and she saw that without an internal object capable of holding the personality together, the infant cannot project into an external object acting as a container. In the absence of this there lies the potential for the personality to liquefy, through dissolution or annihilation, and leak into a limitless space. Bick likened this experience to that of a newborn.

> When a baby is born he is in the position of an astronaut who has been shot out into outer space without a space suit.
>   . . . [T]he predominant terror of the baby is of falling to pieces or liquefying. One can see this in the infant trembling and quivering when the nipple is taken out of his mouth, but also when his clothes are taken off. [1986, p. 66 herein]

What she describes here is an infant without primary skin contain-ment, and it is an extremely dangerous state. One might say that it is almost emotionally fatal. Hence Bick's earlier comment on the franticness of the search for a substitute object cannot be over-emphasized. However, it is also dangerous in terms of further development. In the absence of the containing object, or if it is pre-cariously established, the infant generates omnipotent phantasies that serve to deny the need for the passive experience of the object:

> Disturbance in the primal skin function can lead to a develop-ment of a "second-skin" formation through which dependence on the object is replaced by a pseudo-independence, by the inappropriate use of certain mental functions, or perhaps in-nate talents, for the purpose of creating a substitute for this skin container function. [1968, p. 56 herein]

Examples of what she means here by "inappropriate use" are the infant's premature development of speech, and a muscular devel-opment so that the body is held deliberately rigid and together. In her work with patients—particularly with "Mary", whom she ana-lysed over many years—Bick began to recognize other behaviours that served the function of "second-skin" formation. Here she rec-ognized the meaning of certain of Mary's behaviours as protection against the fear of an experience of separation that would other-wise feel like a laceration. Indeed, from Mary she learnt about what she termed adhesive identification, the "sticking to" quality of secondary skin formation. She developed this concept through working with children who had not introjected a containing object and therefore had no internal space. This "sticking to" objects, a characteristic of autistic children, was therefore seen as a response to the absence of spaces to project into.

When the nipple in the mouth closes the hole in the skin, and an internal space is thus felt, it is clear that the way is paved for object relations to develop. In this, Bick follows Freud in seeing that, from its earliest development, the ego is object-related. This is the same position that Bion took in recognizing that the first object is one that receives primitive communications from the infant, brought about by projective identification. Bick, however, was describing a situation prior to that observed by Freud and Bion.

As is clear from the above, Bick recognized that the capacity to generate phantasies of a containing space is acquired through contact with the object. This is initially a passive experience, for it relies on skin contact. It is also a bodily felt experience. Because the experience of an object that holds the personality together comes through skin and mouth sensations, the first internal object is a bodily felt presence, and primitive communication is a bodily felt phenomenon. With this in mind one can begin to map out a context for some of the clinical chapters in this book. In these, an aspect of bodily experience is observed and thought about in terms of the consequences of there being no object to give a sense of a containment.

The influences on contemporary thinking of these four papers are manifold. Always striving for meaning, and never taking behaviour at face value, Bick helps us to keep looking further beneath the surface. This is the beauty of the observational method, for it allows things to emerge that would not otherwise be seen. The richness of the material presented in the subsequent chapters, whether by clinician, observer, or researcher, demonstrates just how valuable Bick's method is to our understanding of psychic phenomena in general and of the inner world of infants and children in particular. Indeed, such material could not have emerged without the observer's "sympathetic receptive intensity" towards the observed.

The chapters in this book

With Bick's papers firmly in mind, the authors in this book bring to our attention, in part II, contemporary developments inspired by her ideas. Some extend her clinical insights on the experience and function of the skin and raise important questions about technique. Others show how her ideas are informing new ways of working within multidisciplinary teams. Several demonstrate that a close focus on the behaviour of infants and of children allows us more clearly to raise questions of risk.

Child psychotherapists and others in the NHS are currently beginning to address new challenges in developing ways of pro-ducing evidence for the effectiveness of their practice. This brings a plethora of interesting, if taxing, problems to do with defining areas of research and designing instruments that enable clear measurement of aspects of clinical work. Infant observation, being based upon standardized procedures and scrupulous record keep-ing, is easily used as a research method. This is explored by Michael Rustin (chapter 15) and is also the basis of the work re-ported by Stephen Briggs (chapter 11). Another new development is the request for child psychotherapists to assess and write reports on children for the court system: Biddy Youell (chapter 7) shows how close observation, with assessors being clear about their re-sponsibilities, can lead to convincing reports. Again, this is a new development emanating from Bick's ideas.

One of the enduring beauties of the infant observation method is its emphasis on the observer using simple language to describe what is seen. The observer's simplicity of description allows the seminar group to see, as nearly as possible, what he or she has seen. This, in turn, leads to the group seeking even greater clarification, which helps the observer think again more deeply about how to describe what he or she has observed, and brings him or her nearer to a moment when clearer and more "real" patterns can emerge in the observation. The process is described here by Jeanne Magagna (chapter 5), who is frank and honest about the preconceptions that Bick helped her to recognize and think about before she went to each of her observations. A similar account is given by Joan Symington (chapter 6), whose experiences of Bick attending to her work are vivid and riveting to read.

Magagna describes in chapter 5 how Bick's detailed questions about the baby's body movements, postures, and facial expressions "act like a zoom lens of a camera to move the baby into very close, clear focus". Magagna was already an experienced child psychotherapist when she approached Bick to supervise what was a post-qualification observation. Bick was at the very end of her career. However, it is clear that she was still extremely focused on her task of making the inner world of the baby ("Eric") more visible to the observer and seminar group. It is also clear that she was very much in touch at the end of her life with the beginning of life for another and, therefore, with the struggles that she had described in her papers. While it is obvious that Bick's main focus was the infant and child, this did not prevent her from having tremendous understanding for, and about, the mother. This can be seen very clearly in Magagna's account—for example, through Bick's attention to the way the baby is held by the mother.

Joan Symington (chapter 6) gives an account of how Bick herself spoke graphically about the concepts that appeared in her four papers. We hear how she focused on the role of the observer and of her identification with the baby and others in the observational setting; how she described the terrible anxiety for the infant who has not been held by the primary skin relationship, and the omnipotence in the development of his own (secondary) skin formation. While this, as with Magagna's material and experiences, makes for very engaging reading and thinking, it is Symington's account of Bick's description of the primitive projective processes that adds most to our understanding of her work. Bick described these processes in such a way that one cannot escape their being part of the sensual domain inhabited by the infant. In this domain, things stick and are sucked in or stuck onto. This sticking is not always in the service of defence, and Symington illustrates this with vivid examples from her baby observation. We also see something of Bick's focus on the baby and mother together as a relationship. This is moving, especially as we begin to recognize how important this observational method is for identifying difficulties in the mother's mind that have consequences for her mental health and that of her infant. This is a very important chapter in helping us think about early intervention in our work with mothers and their babies.

Since Bick's time, child mental health services have seen a rapid growth in the referrals of children who have suffered emotional, physical or sexual abuse, and various forms of neglect. These children often appear to the outside world to be coping, but careful observation reveals that their apparently ordinary behaviour can have quite different meanings. This is a major theme in Biddy Youell's chapter.

Biddy Youell (chapter 7) discusses her experiences of work in a specialist family centre whose task is the assessment and treatment of families with very young children where there are serious child-protection concerns. One aspect of the work is to assess the parents' potential for change in their capacity to parent their children. The centre's multidisciplinary team have been trained in Bick's method of observation. This is an extremely valuable skill to have in common. Splitting is an ever-present feature of work with children and families where abuse, or allegations of it, have occurred. It is clear that this approach enables each member of the team, having had the opportunity to reflect on what has been observed, to contribute to a clearer understanding of the parenting and other issues that have emerged. This chapter also demonstrates how observational material can be a powerful tool in court reports. When well prepared, this material gives a fresh perspective on a case, revealing the worker's engagement with a baby's or child's world, from which new understandings can be shared about the child's individual responses to his experiences. Its strength in court is enhanced when presented as part of a body of evidence that includes outcome studies.

Jeanne Magagna presents a different account of using Bick's ideas in a collaborative way with colleagues. In her chapter on eating disorders in children diagnosed with pervasive refusal (chapter 8), she introduces her concept of the blockading thumb. These children appear to have given up on life and to want to die. Magagna recognizes that the blockading thumb is the infant's self-protection against what is perceived to be the threat of annihilation. This consists, at various times, of five primitive processes: massive denial, bodily constriction, erotization, omniscience, omnipotence, and adherence to pathological parts of the self. Thus conceptualized, the idea of the blockading thumb takes into account the child's agency. This is of enormous help to those who are trying to help this kind of child to re-establish a link with an object. Magagna describes her approach to reaching these children as being based on Bick's observational method. Its main difference is that Magagna's colleagues and the child's carers are themselves included as observers and, through this, as active agents in the child's treatment. It is this ground-breaking technique that enables carers and workers consistently to provide understanding at the deepest levels of the child's barricaded infantile emotions. In this way the child's anxieties about having a human meeting point can be alleviated.

R. D. Hinshelwood (chapter 9) describes another creative adaptation of Bick's infant observation method. He applied the technique to the training of psychiatrists, who undertook observations on a psychiatric back-ward to observe relationships between staff and residents. The aim was twofold. First, that through observing the culture of the ward trainees would begin to understand something about their own culture, and some of the emotional attitudes and values into which they are inducted by joining their profession. Second, in observing how staff performed the ward's task to care for patients, trainees could attempt to understand the staff's emotional responses to this task and factors that might prevent it from being carried out fully. Hinshelwood describes an observation by one of his trainees and reveals how Bick's method has generated material that sheds new light on the findings of studies outside its original, infant and family, setting. Here he includes, among others, Goffman (1961), Jaques (1953, 1955), Menzies (1959), and Trist (1950).

Jan Dollery introduces in chapter 10 another new application of Bick's ideas, in discussing her experiences within a very different work setting. My collaboration with this chapter came after several years of reflecting informally with her on the interesting and difficult work she does teaching children from a Traveller community. In using observational skills from the Tavistock model, she has developed further insights about children and families in a culture that few child psychotherapists or other professionals are currently likely to meet in their work. Her thesis is that, while there is copious evidence that Traveller infants may have an experience of what

Bick referred to as nipple in mouth, or primary skin, containment, it is also clear that this is a very fragile skin that needs a secondary formation in order for the infant to survive.

While her observations of the children lead her to wonder about the nature of their attachments, her thinking also extends to the nature of the parents' attachment to their culture. This attachment appears to be largely adhesive. Dollery suggests that, while there is strong evidence that Traveller children are held in mind by their parents, this may be similar to the experience of being held by a secondary skin formation. Using very graphic material she shows that her work with these young children suggests that they have well-developed secondary skins. This way of relating to the world is reinforced by the culture that also holds their parents together. Such is the importance of this culture that it takes very powerful events in a family's life to shake the function it holds for them. However, it does not stay shaken for long, as observation reveals that the individuals involved have very limited capacities to process these events, and therefore the skin rapidly slips over the wound they have caused, covering up its effects .

Traveller children are a new group for child mental health and other professional workers to read about. To speculate on the possibility of offering any form of intervention to children from such a closed group requires us first to think about the implications of observing cross-culturally. This sort of observation raises a number of important issues. One is of understanding the beliefs and behaviours of another culture, and this is recognized in Dollery's chapter. Another, and related to this, is how an observer from within a host, settled, or dominant culture positions him/herself in a family from a different ethnic group. In chapter 11, Stephen Briggs revisits his study of infants at risk and discusses some of the fraught experiences he met with in his observation of a baby boy in a Bengali family.

Briggs's account of observing Hashmat, the ninth child in a Bengali family, makes for painful reading. We follow Briggs's analysis of his observational material, generated to give a "multi-layered" understanding of processes developing into emotional risk for this baby boy. However, while this gives us a harrowing view of Hashmat's development within this particular environment, which leaves him fighting for his emotional and physical survival, it simultaneously raises a very important question about cross-cultural studies of this kind. Hashmat's parents spoke very little English, and they firmly maintained a traditional way of life. The limits this put on verbal communication between family and observer, and the observer's imperative to suspend judgement in the collection of material, all led to particular difficulties for Briggs. Not least, he needed to rely on nonverbal observation to understand risk. Also, given that the concept of risk is generated in one culture about the child-care activities of another, he needed to struggle hard to be clearer about the specific qualities of the situation he was looking at. The problem of whether, and how much, a child is at risk within its own ethnic culture is a question that all child workers are faced with today. Through repeated, painstaking observations Briggs began to recognize risk regardless of culture. His struggle with these difficulties has yielded for us a rich opportunity to learn from his experience.

Esther Bick believed that the presence of the observer is likely to have a therapeutic effect on the family, largely through his or her capacity to bear their projections. This effect can be seen in Briggs's role as observer—for example, when he records that Rani, Hashmat's mother, began to watch his play "benignly, and with interest". Similar effects are evident in Dollery's chapter. Although her role was as a teacher rather than as an observer, her ability to bear and contain projections facilitated significant emotional development in the children she worked with. The therapeutic effect also appears throughout Magagna's observation of Eric. This effect is often brought about through being able to bear intense anxieties on the family's behalf, which offers the observer the opportunity to learn something from what has been projected. This is very evident in the chapter on the observation of baby "Peter" by Judith Jackson and Eleanor Nowers.

Jackson and Nowers (chapter 12) describe a harrowing observation. Peter's mother loved but misunderstood him and did not seem to be aware that as a result her baby was suffering. She saw him as a contented baby, whereas the observer saw him as a baby who had begun to develop severe physical skin problems. Soon he was scratching and twisting his skin in a way that prompted the observer to wonder whether he was "creating a bodily experience of being both the container of the body and also the contained".

Certainly, it soon appeared that this activity was in the service of the denial of dependence and deprivation and had become a perversion. With great relief, one eventually reads of Peter's father rescuing both Peter and his mother from this painful situation and taking on a crucial role in Peter's development. Being released from this destructive relationship between himself and his mother enabled Peter to develop his motor skills, which had been held back by the "invisible bonds" that his secondary skin activities had, in effect, become. Another fascinating aspect of this observation is that the observer was able to meet Peter again when he was 10 years old. This provided an illustration of Bick's view that faulty skin formation produces general fragility in later integration. Again, this has implications for the current research agenda for child psychotherapists and other professionals, and one thinks of the importance of infant observation in longitudinal studies.

The close attention to detail through observation, and the capacity to bear projections as well as one's own anxieties, are central to the work of the child psychotherapist. Being able to explore these experiences in one's own mind allows for more accurate words to form, prior to making an intervention in clinical work. Bick did not address issues surrounding this kind of intervention in her papers. In their contributions to this collection, Maria Rhode and Anne Alvarez both discuss intervention in their work with very damaged and disturbed children.

Rhode's discussion (chapter 13) is of her highly original work with children who have difficulties in recognizing that self and object must be appropriately separate. One of the children she presents is Clara, a child who exemplifies the confusion of ownership inherent in Bick's adhesive identification. Clara, like the other children, has difficulty realizing that the contact point between her skin and her mother's skin marks the boundary of her separate body. This boundary, representing the fact of physical separateness from the mother, may be seen by the infant as the cause of any pain he suffers. Sometimes the baby and mother can be thought of as competing for the skin as something essential, which protects them and makes them feel complete.

Taking us further into the sensory world explored by Bick, Rhode draws a parallel between mental and sensual containment. She develops Bick's implication that the mother's skin is the physical counterpart of the psychic processes described by Bion. The emphasis here is on the mother's ability to tolerate and process aspects of the infant's personality, which allows the infant to feel that a skin holds parts of his personality together. This is both physical and psychic. Thus, according to Rhode, "failures in emotional interaction will all have correlates in terms of how the child experiences his own skin in relation to the skin boundary of the mother". The problem of possession poses great technical difficulties for the psychotherapist, who is effectively working with children whose identities have become confused. Interpretations can be felt by the child as being addressed to their physical skin, thus activating a sensual response. In this way the psychotherapist's interpretations, being received by the child as sensual experiences, can be felt as part of the child's self. This links with the difficulty the child has in recognizing the psychotherapist as separate.

The technical difficulties of working with children whose development has been seriously impaired through their adherence to secondary skin formation are of particular interest to Anne Alvarez (chapter 14). She discusses ways of reaching these children and uses her knowledge of developmental psychology to think about aspects of technique while recognizing that such adhesion has severe consequences.

Alvarez explores the problem of reaching children who have developmental problems arising from difficulties in their early relationship with their mothers. Through a discussion of what she sees as the difference between animate and inanimate, stuck and unstuck, she emphasizes the need for work with autistic children to be developmentally as well as psychoanalytically informed. Through her use of the animate technique, Alvarez demonstrates the possibility of developing thinking for the stuck and inanimate children she discusses. Alvarez sees children like those described by Bick as not so much in fear of disintegration but, rather, in a state of unformation. Central to her technique for helping these children is Bion's idea that in order to link, the child needs a concept of an object that can be relied upon for this function. She discusses how what she terms the drawing of unformed, unmantled personalities relies upon the object to begin the process that leads to the child becoming drawn, mantled, and formed. This involves the development of a space in which thought is possible and a mind can be formed. Alvarez seems to be suggesting that thinking may not be possible for children with the Bick defence, but that it may be developed with the help of a psychotherapist, whose skill is to draw the child's personality outside its skin and to let the child see what is being drawn and how this is being done. These complex questions have many implications for how we understand Bick children, and how we conceptualize their treatment.

In the final chapter of the book, Michael Rustin, in recognizing the contribution of Bick's method to research in psychoanalysis, further develops an area he has been exploring for some years. Rustin's chapter could be described in simple terms as bringing together the psychoanalytic thinking of Freud with that of Bick. Freud left his followers with a body of theory largely based on a Hegelian model of causality. Bick, even more than Mrs Klein, moved psychoanalytic thinking further towards the hermeneutic approach, allowing complexity as an intrinsic part of understanding the meanings of patterns and less precise phenomena in clinical and research settings. In this way, meanings and intentions are allowed to be free of any attempt to impose a meaningful context for them that has been defined by a perceived cause.

This said, Rustin argues for the importance of both meaning and causality in psychoanalysis, and he suggests that a way out of the dichotomy this presents for researchers is through complexity theory. Complexity theory recognizes that a large area of nature is not subject either to patterned or random ways of behaving. Linking this to psychoanalysis, Rustin says: "The assumption of complexity theory that realities are complex, emergent, non-reversible over time, and liable to generate increased difference is consistent with both the humanistic and the scientific assumptions of psychoanalysis." One example here could be Bick's concept of secondary skin formation. If this were treated as a research hypothesis of complexity theory, and tested against evidence, many different types of secondary skin formation might be found in exactly the ways that complexity theory would anticipate, described by Rustin as "self-organizing systems, of high complexity, and indeterminacy within understood limits ". Rustin's chapter is particularly important for child psychotherapists and other mental health professionals who are struggling to find ways to research the effectiveness of their practice. However, it goes further than this, helping us to think about how to present and report our findings in contexts outside the clinical setting, without compromising their meaning.

* * *

Esther Bick saw infant observation as a process of discovery. Through this one waits for things to emerge, so that they can then be seen and understood more clearly for what they are. Her own use of this method allowed her to illuminate the struggle for psychic survival experienced by every infant. Her description of infants for whom this struggle is fraught by difficult relations with their objects is particularly graphic. Her papers have proved inspirational both for subsequent generations of child psychotherapists and for many other professions, who have used them as part of a training in infant observation to extend their understanding of the complex world of infants and their families. It is now time to read her papers and the other chapters in this book.

PART I

PIONEERING IDEAS:
THE PAPERS OF ESTHER BICK

CHAPTER ONE

Child analysis today

[1962]

This Symposium is in the nature of an historical event—it is the first symposium on child analysis at an International Congress of Psycho-Analysis. In May 1927, such a symposium was held before the British Psycho-Analytical Society. On that occasion Melanie Klein contrasted the development of child analysis with that of adult analysis, discussing the striking fact that although child analysis had a history of about eighteen years, its fundamental principles had not yet been clearly enunciated, whereas, after a similar period in the history of adult analysis, the basic principles had been laid down, empirically tested, and the fundamental principles of technique firmly established. She went on to discuss why the analysis of children had been so much less fortunate in its development.

I am well aware that progress has been made during the last thirty-four years, both in actual child analysis and in its allied fields, such as in Child Guidance Clinics, progress which has been deeply and variously influenced by the work of Melanie Klein and

Read at the 22nd International Psycho-Analytical Congress, Edinburgh, July–August 1961.

Anna Freud. To give examples, the range of children who are felt to be suitable for treatment has been extended: play technique is now in general use, though often in a modified form; the importance of interpretations has been widely accepted, and there is a greater recognition of the psycho-analytic approach in the training of child psychotherapists and child psychiatrists.

However, if we examine the position of child analysis in relation to the whole field of psycho-analysis, we see what a small place it occupies in terms of practice of child analysis, of training, of scientific discussions and publications. Very few people trained in adult analysis go on to train as child analysts, and very few institutes of psycho-analysis are able to offer systematic training in child analysis, the British Institute being the only one, I believe, to give an actual qualification. Even this training is recognized to be inadequate. Contributions from child analysts to scientific discussions are numerically very low—for example, less than 5% of papers at International Congress are on child cases.

This neglect of child analysis is the more striking when we consider the vital interest of analysts in the psychology of children as a source of understanding of emotional development and our concern about the prophylactic aspects of child analysis. The position of psycho-analysis in the community must also to a great extent depend on its offering help to children and its understanding of their emotional problems.

There must, therefore, be specific difficulties interfering with the development of child analysis which do not apply to the same extent to adult analysis. In this paper I shall attempt to contribute to the understanding of this problem. In order to do so, I shall discuss some of the differences between analysing adults and analysing children, from the point of view both of the student and of the practising analyst. I shall discuss the stresses and gratifications, both external and internal.

First, to consider some of the external stresses: the student who is embarking on child analysis may be restricted owing to commitments related to his training in adult analysis, both financially and with regard to the times he has available, which may not suit the child's parents. There is also the difficulty for the student that the ordinary parent will only undertake to bring the child five times a week over a period of years if the child is severely ill, and such cases are not suitable for the beginner in child analysis.

An analyst wanting to restrict himself to child analysis would find it unrewarding financially. Certain aspects of child analysis, such as keeping in contact with the parents and caring for the playroom, can be very time consuming. These are real difficulties, but they can be used as rationalizations to cover up the emotional problems of studying and practising child analysis.

Before discussing the emotional stresses, however, it is important to remember the pleasures and gratifications arising out of child analysis, such as the unique opportunity for intimate contact with primitive layers of the child's unconscious mind; the sense of privilege in being entrusted by the parents with their child; the awareness that one is dealing with a human being who has almost all his life ahead of him and who is still in the early stages of developing his potentialities.

I want now to turn to the internal stresses, and shall divide these into two categories: first, those which are in the nature of pre-formed anxieties related to the treatment of children as such, and second, the specific counter-transference problems. In the first category there are the student's general anxieties about his ability to communicate with children, especially if he has had little or no previous experience with young children. There are also the anxieties about taking responsibility. These are much greater with children than with adults, not only because it is a dual responsibility—to the child as well as to his parents—but also because the less mature the patient's ego, the greater is the responsibility resting on the analyst.

The student has to be clear about what his responsibility is in analysing the child, although this may clash with what he feels the parents really want of him. Here belongs, for example, the responsibility of analysing such problems as the child's hostility and his sexual wishes towards the parents. This may provoke anxiety in the student concerning his relation with the parents. Closely associated with this is the question of setting independently, on the basis of one's clinical judgement, aims for the analysis, as distinct from aiming to cure the presenting symptoms for which the child was originally brought for treatment. There are also anxieties related to becoming excessively attached to, or hurtful to, the child. The former anxiety may lead to greater strictness, to a type of behaviour which interferes with the unfolding of the positive transference. The latter anxiety may lead to reassurance, to a denial of the child's hostile feelings and persecutory anxiety, or to such behaviour as appealing to the child's reason—suggesting that the analyst has been unable to accept painful analytical responsibility and has assumed the role of parent substitute.

Such anxieties, related to the painful aspects of responsibility, may be kept within bounds and often diminished through the help of a supervisor who shares the responsibility. But if they are too severe, they can impose such grave limitations on therapeutic effectiveness that supervision can be of little or no help and only further analysis can enable the student to overcome the inhibiting unconscious conflicts. Such anxieties approximate to those of the second category, the stresses arising out of countertransference phenomena.

As Freud stated in 1910: "We have become aware of the counter-transference, which arises in him (the physician) as a result of the patient's influence on his unconscious feelings. . . . We have noticed that no psycho-analyst goes further than his own complexes and internal resistances permit" [1910d]. I have suggested that the counter-transference stresses on the child analyst are more severe than those on the analyst of adults, at any rate of non-psychotic adults. This is due, I think, to two specific factors: first, the unconscious conflicts which arise in relation to the child's parents; and second, the nature of the child's material.

With regard to the first factor, the child analyst has the constant problem of his unconscious identifications. He may identify with the child against the parents, or with the parents against the child, or with a protective parental attitude towards the child. These conflicts often lead to a persecutory and guilty attitude towards the parents, making the analyst over-critical of them and over-dependent on their approval. In addition, there is the student's difficulty in understanding the twofold nature of the child's relationship to his parents: his normal and healthy dependence on them, relative to his age, and the infantile elements in the relationship, due to his internal difficulties. The more this is recognized and accepted by the student, the more the infantile parts of the child can come into the transference, with a resulting improvement in his relationship to his parents, even in the early months of analysis. The student can then foresee and be prepared for the risk that the parents will lose sight of the child's illness and want to stop treatment, and for an intensification of difficulties at home during analytic holidays.

I cannot go into the many vicissitudes of the analyst's difficulties in his relationship with the parents. It is an integral part of his work, intricate and delicate to handle, needing flexibility and considerable confidence in child analysis in general and one's own work in particular. If one can take these things for granted, the relationship with many parents can become an added source of gratification.

The second specific factor in child analysis concerns the strain imposed on the mental apparatus of the analyst, both by the content of the child's material and its mode of expression. The intensity of the child's dependence, of his positive and negative transference, the primitive nature of his phantasies, tend to arouse the analyst's own unconscious anxieties. The violent and concrete projections of the child into the analyst may be difficult to contain. Also the child's suffering tends to evoke the analyst's parental feelings, which have to be controlled so that the proper analytic role can be maintained. All these problems tend to obscure the analyst's understanding and to increase in turn his anxiety and guilt about his work.

Moreover, the child's material may be more difficult to understand than the adult's, since it is more primitive in its sources as well as in its mode of expression, and requires a deeper knowledge of the primitive levels of the unconscious. One may have to sit with children for a long time completely in the dark about what is going on, until suddenly something comes up from the depth that illuminates it, and one interprets without always being able to see how one reached that conclusion. It imposes on the child analyst a greater dependence on his unconscious to provide him with clues to the meaning of the child's play and non-verbal communications.

I will bring two clinical examples to illustrate some of the points I have made. The first concerns a case of my own, the second, one of an analyst supervised by me. I am giving an instance from a first session of a nine-year-old boy, referred on account of bed wetting, shyness, and clinging to his mother. He came into the treatment room with me and stood twisting his cap and blushing. I pointed out that he might feel awkward because he might not know what we were going to do here. There was no response. I showed him his box with play material and said that was for his use in the sessions. He made no movement but stood there as if dazed. I said that he had been told that he would be coming to see me five times a week, and that I would try to help him with his worries; but it seemed to me that he expected something quite different which he was not able to tell me or might not even know himself. He continued his silence and immobility, but looked tense and troubled. Then he glanced towards the paper on the table. I said that he indicated he would find it easier to tell me something on paper than to talk. He nodded, sat down, and drew a hut on the mountains, a path, and a tree. When I asked him about this, he told me it was about a young man who lived alone in a log cabin in the mountains. He had a deer who kept him company. One night a man came and stole the deer. When the young man woke in the morning he could not find the deer. He went out of the cabin and saw the tracks of a man and of his deer in the snow. He followed the tracks. He was afraid that the man might kill him, but he went on. He told me this story in a solemn, dull way. I said that there was a Christmas tree in the drawing, and that in this way he was telling me one of the things he expected from me: that I should be like Father Christmas who would make everything wonderful, and that perhaps he had waited for the analysis as he had waited for Father Christmas as a small boy. He smiled, his whole face lit up, and he said: "Fancy you should say that! This morning a boy at school asked me if a fairy told me I could have three wishes what would I want."

I interpreted that we could now understand why he could not speak at the beginning of the session. On the one hand he hoped that he would find in me a fairy capable of fulfilling all his wishes in a magic way; at the same time he was afraid that I might be a witch who would cast a spell on him and immobilize him; it seemed that he had felt this when he could neither move nor speak at the beginning of the session. In the story there were two male figures: one was Father Christmas, and the other the man who stole his deer and might kill him. So as with the fairy and the witch he also hoped that I might be a father who, like Father Christmas, would give him what he wanted most—to keep his deer forever.

But he was also afraid that I might be like the man who would steal it from him. Such were his hopes and fears before he came, and when he met me, he did not know which of the figures I was. Although he was very frightened, he came with me into the room, perhaps thinking that if he did what I wanted, I would not harm him; and also because he so much wanted help in tracking down his worries and becoming cured.

He said, "Yes, I didn't tell the boy that my wish would be to be cured from bed wetting, I can't do anything, I can't go camping with the Scouts. I can't stop it." We then went on to the other important meanings of the deer.

What can be seen in this boy, as in many other young patients, is that, together with the hope of finding a solution to his internal problems, there is also a deep pessimism about being understood by the adult world. This can be seen clearly in the boy's excitement when he exclaimed, "Fancy you should say that!"

My second example is taken from the first session of a three-year-old girl. She followed the analyst stiffly but easily into the play-room. He told her that the toys on the table and in the drawer were for her to play with. She looked into the drawer, took out a toy sheep, sat down and began to handle the pencil. The analyst asked whether it was a mummy, a daddy, or a baby sheep; but this made her increasingly withdrawn. She began to rock and suck a sweet she had in her mouth. The analyst interpreted her feeling of being alone and frightened and her wish to be with her Mummy, and linked it with her feeling at night and a wish to snuggle up and have her bottle with Mummy. Her head dropped, there was some play with her fingers of the "little piggy" type. The analyst indicated to her her wish for Mummy's soft breast to sleep on. Her head dropped and hit the table. The analyst put a pillow there. Her head drooped backwards, and he put the pillow behind her, but she systematically avoided it. He interpreted that the pillow was unable to replace Mummy's breast, and her similar discomfort and dis-satisfaction with the analyst. There was some rubbing of eyes, scratching of the face, and picking of the nose. The analyst interpreted her disappointment in having a man as an analyst and suggested she had hoped to have a woman, like her brother who was also in analysis. He also indicated it was about time to stop. She gave the sheep back to him, looked at him, and seemed in fair contact with him before leaving. In the following session there was a marked change in the nature of the contact with the analyst. She produced rich detailed material in which her anxieties about the transference to him as the brother came to the fore.

We see in the opening session with the little girl how what seemed to be very sparse material became richer and more detailed following interpretations; whereas in the case of the older boy, material rich in detail but impoverished of emotion became flooded with feeling and contact through interpretation. In both cases the interpretations were based initially on the analyst's intuitive response to the situation growing out of the pre-verbal projective process from the child's unconscious into the analyst. In the case of the little girl, the sleeping and the near falling had the effect of projecting into the analyst considerable anxiety for her safety, which he actually dealt with by providing her with a real pillow. Her systematic avoidance of the pillow increased his feeling of hopelessness to protect her. These two projections worked together: "I cannot help this child; in fact I will damage her because I have not got the right kind of pillow." It was not until the interpretation of her disappointment in the analyst as a man, without real breasts, that she came into contact with the analyst on leaving and produced the enriched material of the next day, expressing her anxiety of repeating with the analyst her sexual involvement with her brother.

In the case of the boy, he conveyed from the beginning his distress through his non-verbal behaviour. The analyst's anxiety led her to give explanations about the analytic procedure. In this situation, these were tantamount to reassurance and therefore made no contact with the child. Following his glance, the analyst invited him to draw. The picture and the story were produced flatly, lifelessly, although the story in itself seemed vital and filled with anxiety. The analyst felt that the hopelessness which he projected into her, both at the beginning of the session and through his lifeless dull way of telling the story, came from a more primitive level than the oedipal material. She reacted to the Christmas tree as representing a far deeper process of splitting his objects into ideally good and dreadfully persecuting ones, with their magic powers for good or evil. She was able to make contact with his primitive internal world of witches and fairies, and in this way to reach the split-off affects of hope for an omnipotent good object.

Thus with both children, following leads from the depths arising from the taking in of projected distress, the analysts were able to interpret into the deeper strata. In the case of the little girl, with regard to her expectations of a real breast to sleep on and suck; in the case of the boy, the hope for an omnipotent fairy to protect him against persecutors.

In addition to the ability to deal with the kind of material that the child spontaneously produces and to bear his concrete projections, there is the difficulty of allowing the child to experience pain without intruding in a non-analytic way. The strain in bearing the child's suffering is greater than with adults, not only because of the child's weaker ego, but because of his appeal to one's parental feelings. This is painful when the child is persecuted or crying, but particularly so when he is trying to be good and repair, but cannot manage it because of internal conflicts. A little girl broke most of the toy figures following the first holiday in the analysis. After some working through of her holiday feelings, she decided to mend the mother figure of which she had broken the head and an arm. She managed with difficulty to stick the head on with Plasticine, but was very clumsy in fixing the arm. It kept falling off. She was very distressed, but persevered for a long time. Eventually she said, pointing to the figure, "She is tired", and gave up. In such a situation the child analyst may find great difficulty in resisting the mute appeal of the child for direct help.

My comments on the internal stresses of the child analyst can perhaps be best summarized by a quotation for Gitelson's paper "The Emotional Position of the Analyst in the Psycho-Analytic Situation" (1949). After quoting Freud's original definition of transference, he goes on to say: "If the transference is to be a truly irrational recapitulation of childhood relationships subject to psycho-analytic interpretation, then nothing in the current reality must intervene to give it concurrent validity. These are still the guiding principles of classical psycho-analytic technique." This quotation refers to adult analysis, Klein was guided by the same principle of classical psycho-analytic technique in her work with children. She showed that in order to do this the child analyst has to provide an analytic setting, both external and within himself, to enable the child to re-experience the irrational infantile and childhood relationships. I have tried to show that it is easier to accept the external setting which Klein evolved in her play technique than to accept and tolerate the stress produced by adhering to the fundamental psycho-analytic attitude in work with child patients.

The student of child analysis is thus exposed to great anxieties. It is, therefore, important that he should do the child training while he is himself in analysis; and, indeed, the working over of these anxieties will help to deepen his analysis. I have found that analysis of children brings a greater conviction to the student about the reality of unconscious phantasy than his work with adults. To see this concretely presented in the child's play and in his spontaneous communications, and to see the immediacy of relief from, or change in the nature of, anxiety following prompt interpretations, constitutes in itself an unending source of wonder and delight to many child analysts.

In conclusion, the aim of this paper is to draw attention to the grave neglect of child analysis. I have singled out two factors responsible for its slow development: the external stresses associated with financial and time difficulties, constantly exacerbated by the lack of adequate training, and the manifold internal stresses which are an integral part of the nature of child analysis. I have also indicated the gratifications inherent in analysing children and have stressed the importance of further developing this work, both in terms of its value to psychoanalytic understanding in general and in its contribution to the community.

CHAPTER TWO

Notes on infant observation in psycho-analytic training

[1964]

I nfant observation was introduced into the curriculum of the Institute of Psycho-Analysis in London in 1960 as part of the course for first year students. The detailed observational mate- rial that I am quoting in this paper is mainly drawn from the work of these students. Infant observation had, in fact, been part of the training course for child psychotherapists at the Tavistock Clinic since 1948 when the course began. We then decided to include in the first non-clinical year some practical experience of infants.

I thought this important for many reasons but, perhaps, mostly because it would help the students to conceive vividly the infantile experience of their child patients, so that when, for example, they started the treatment of a two-and-a-half-year-old child they would get the feel of the baby that he was and from which he is not so far removed. It should also increase the student's understanding of the child's non-verbal behaviour and his play, as well as the behaviour of the child who neither speaks nor plays. Further, it should help the student when he interviews the mother and enable

---

A paper read to the British Psycho-Analytical Society, July 1963.

him to understand better her account of the child's history. It would also give each student a unique opportunity to observe the development of an infant more or less from birth, in his home setting and in his relation to his immediate family, and thus to find out for himself how these relations emerge and develop. In addition he would be able to compare and contrast his observations with those of his fellow students in the weekly seminars.

I want to turn now to the method of observation which has evolved over the years and has been constantly discussed in seminars. The child psychotherapy students visit the family once a week up to about the end of the second year of the child's life, each observation normally lasting about an hour. The observations of the candidates at the Institute usually stop at about the end of the first year. Contrary to our expectations, there was no difficulty in finding mothers willing to have an observer—either through acquaintances or through other channels. Mothers have frequently indicated explicitly or implicitly how much they welcomed the fact of having someone come regularly into their home with whom they could talk about their baby and its development and their feelings about it. We found that it was best to give a simple explanation to the parents—namely, that the observer wished to have some direct experience of babies as part of his professional development. Note-taking during the observation was soon recognized as unsuitable and disturbing as it interfered with free-floating attention and prevented the student from responding easily to the emotional demands of the mother.

Much thought had to be given to the central problem of the role of the observer in the whole situation. This problem seemed to be twofold, as it involved the conceptualization of the observer's role, and also the conscious and unconscious attitudes of the observer. First the question of role; as infant observation was planned as an adjunct to the teaching of psycho-analysis and child therapy, rather than as a research instrument, it was felt to be important that the observer should feel himself sufficiently inside the family to experience the emotional impact, but not committed to act out any roles thrust upon him, such as giving advice or registering approval or disapproval. This would not seem to exclude him being helpful as a particular situation arose—by holding the baby, or bringing it an

occasional gift. In other words, he would be a privileged and therefore grateful participant observer.

The second problem, that of attitudes, is, however, more difficult. Here, in the house of parents with a newborn baby, the observer, however experienced with babies or in psycho-analysis or
in scientific methods of observation, is confronted with a situation
of intense emotional impact. In order to be able to observe at all he
must attain detachment from what is going on. Yet he must, as in
the basic method of psycho-analysis, find a position from which to
make his observations, a position that will introduce as little distortion as possible into what is going on in the family. He has to allow
some things to happen and to resist others. Rather than actively
establishing his own personality as a new addition to the family
organization he has to allow the parents, particularly the mother,
to fit him into her household in her own way. But he must resist
being drawn into roles involving intense infantile transference and
therefore counter-transference.

To give an example, an older child in the family may try to
monopolize him as an ally against the mother–baby couple. The
mother may attempt to build up a strong dependence relation. He
may find himself being influenced by the baby to become a substitute mother. In other words, if he becomes involved in the family
organization as do other members of the family—grandparents,
father, relatives, friends, who all "observe" after all—his observations would then be as little objective as those of a father or mother
student wanting to bring observations of their own. Further the
tensions of the situation would invade him; particularly, the inad-
equacies in the care of the infant would upset him and the whole
mystery of the situation intrigue him too much. He must not allow
his behaviour to be dominated by these feelings which, on close
scrutiny, will often be found to have been intensified by projections
from members of the family. While much of this must be dealt with
in the student's analysis, the seminar can at least uncover some of
the projections into him that are operating and which intensify his
own internal conflicts.

To illustrate this function of the seminar I have chosen for discussion a problem which has appeared the most ubiquitous and
difficult, namely the operation of the mother's post-partum depres-

sive trends. While we have known for some time that these trends are almost universal, I was not prepared for the intensity with which they impinged on the observer. What one was struck by was the exclusive preoccupation of the students in the seminar with the mother's handling of the baby. Their attitude was highly critical and emotional. At first I tried to mitigate the problem by encouraging them to give more attention to the baby and less to the mother. This did not help. I realized it was necessary to give more consideration to this factor—the depression in the mother and its impact on the observer as well as on the baby and other members of the family. It is, of course, not the purpose of this paper to attempt to give a systematic account of depression in the mothers of newborn babies, but before giving the observational reports I want to clarify how I am using the word "depressive" here. I am not using it primarily descriptively, but rather metapsychologically, to describe those aspects of the mother's relation to the baby in which a clear-cut regression to part-object relationship is evident. The mother can be clearly seen to be experiencing emotional detachment from the baby, helplessness in understanding and meeting its needs, relying on the baby to make use of her breasts, hands, voice, as part-objects.

Naturally depressive trends tend strongly to disturb the observer's detachment, both because of the mother's needs which pull the observer, and counter-transference anxieties which push him. He is pulled towards augmenting the mother's vitality and pushed to identify with the disturbed and resentful aspects of the baby. To illustrate this problem of the way in which the mother's postpartum depressive trends tend to draw the observer into roles unsuitable to his function and to place him under greater emotional stress, I will bring two different types of material: one, a summary of two months' observational work, and the second, more detailed observational notes. I think in both examples one can feel the observer's struggle to tolerate the situation. In the first example it will be seen how the crumbling of the manic trends in the mother tends to draw the observer into the role of a dependent figure.

K., a male baby, was the first child of young parents (about 25 years old) who worked together as office caretakers. The baby was unplanned and came after two years of marriage. Some months later, when the mother was much more secure about herself as a mother, she confessed to the observer that when other girls at school had talked of getting married and having children she thought privately to herself: "Married may be, but I'll never have a baby; I am sure I should let it die." This mother was specially selected by a health visitor as one who was normal, capable, and unlikely to be disturbed by being observed. The mother continued work up to term despite diarrhoea and backache, as part of her dependent and grateful relationship to her devoted husband. She described the rather precipitous delivery which had caused her some lacerations as a delivery in which, once his head was through, "he shot out". Thus she expressed an attitude emphasizing the baby's strength and independence which she maintained later.

At the first observation, when the baby was two days old, mother and baby were enthroned amid flowers, presents, and new furnishings; the mother, radiant, talked incessantly in an excited way about her pride in the baby, her delight that he was a boy and so strong, the presents she had received, and her gratitude to her husband who helped her so much in the last weeks. At the same time she was planning to fit the baby into a routine which would enable her to go on with her work and to help her husband. She reiterated her intention to breast-feed, driven by the conviction that it produced less flabby babies, but she was plainly very uncertain about her ability to do so.

Five days later all was changed. The mother was up, tired and harassed-looking, feeling burdened by the observer's visit but impelled to incessant talk. She said she had never thought that feeding a baby and keeping him clean would take up so much time, or that it would take so much to satisfy him. She had a blister on her nipple and pains under her arm, and talked in terms of trying to continue breast-feeding for six weeks.

When the baby who had been asleep in the pram, began to cry, the mother seemed at a loss to comfort him, talking rapidly to the observer of his strength, the beauty of the pram, and of her overworked state. Finally, she turned the baby over, saying, "Mustn't spoil you, young man", and told the observer that though they had not specially wanted a baby she and her husband were quite delighted, but since she had never much liked other people's babies she did not know what to do with him, and ended, "I've really let myself in for something now."

Further observations in the early weeks were similar, as the mother struggled to satisfy this "wild, hungry baby", as she called him, who strained so hard both to get at and get away from the breast, who wanted but seemed unable to get all "the dark part of the nipple into his mouth", who wriggled and struggled when being changed, quite unlike the doll they practised on in the ante-natal clinic. She continued to try to comfort him in the pram, to dress and undress him on the table. When the baby was screaming with hunger and impatience after the bath she would go on talking while dressing him in an apparently unconcerned way. At other times, when the baby was distressed, she pressed him on the ob-server while she got on with other tasks or even while she chatted. The breast-feeding ended at six weeks.

The father seemed to give the mother a great deal of support; he sometimes impersonated the baby to express gentle criticism of the mother or to indicate the baby's feelings to her. He did not compete with her in her role as mother, he regarded her unquestioningly, despite all her uncertainties, as the expert as far as the baby was concerned, and was at hand whenever possible. This supportive behaviour of the father seemed to be an important factor in the gradual improvement in the mother's closeness and tolerance to-wards the baby. In this material the manic defences of an immature and dependent mother can be seen to collapse, revealing her great anxiety about being able to take care of the baby and her distrust in her ability to do so.

The observer's anxiety about the inadequacy of this baby's mothering comes through in her difficulty in tolerating such points as the mother's incessant talking when the baby was in distress and the mother's lack of warmth and concern for her baby, as well as in her own relief at the father's support and its effect on the family. The seminar also felt that as the relationship between mother and observer went on there were indications of a helpful improvement, evidenced, for example, in the mother's being able to tell the ob-server of her adolescent anxieties about ever being able to be a mother at all.

In the second example I will give an account of a first observa-tion, both to show the observer at work, indicating, as I said earlier on, the impact of the mother's depression on him, and also to show the richness of observational data—a point to which I shall come back later.

Charles, a baby of ten days at the first observation, was the second child of a professional couple. I shall quote now from the report.

"I rang mother and explained who I was in terms of the line of contact and we arranged that I should come the next day so that we could meet and see how we liked each other and whether we could make an arrangement for observations. In fixing the time of this meeting mother asked whether I would like to see the baby awake or didn't it matter. When I said I would prefer to see the baby awake, she suggested a feed, which I took up very readily. She showed some eagerness to accommodate me, being prepared to move the time of the feed up to half an hour. I said I could come when he was usually fed.

"Mother is aged about 25, has glasses, short thick light-brown hair, a square masculine sort of head and face, rather quiet and serious in looks and voice, but smiles readily with a warm smile. She was wearing a Swedish-Liberty striped blouse and a large black skirt; rather shabby-looking was the general impression, but somehow not in an unattractive way. She had quite a dignified manner, although visibly anxious about how to deal with me.

"I was first taken out to the garden behind the house where the mother's mother sat holding Charles wrapped in a blanket. The mother muttered something about it being feeding-time and would I care to see the feed. I followed her and Charles back into the living-room. The mother sat first on a divan and invited me to pull up an armchair opposite, then changed places because there was a draught on to the divan from the door to the garden (and grandma). By changing places the door could be left open without any draught on her. It also meant that the mother could be seen by her mother from the garden. While the divan where I sat could not.

"When I first saw Charles he was wrapped very voluminously in the blanket on his grandmother's lap. When the blanket was drawn back he was lying with his left hand on his ear, his right hand over the whole front of his face, kneading his cheeks and mouth and nose. His right thumb was in his mouth. He had several scratches on his cheeks and upper cheekbone and his right eye

looked faintly discoloured, as though he had poked it too hard.
When the mother and Charles settled in the armchair for the feed I
could see very little of him indeed. I asked his name and how old
he was. The mother asked me about my work. I explained that I
hoped to work with children ultimately. We discussed possible
times for me to come, and the mother seemed to prefer me to come
to see the bath rather than a feed. This, however, was a misunderstanding. We found a suitable time and agreed that arrangements
would be flexible because Charles's time-table would change and
we could see how things went. Mother apologized for the unfinished state of the house, pointing out the packing-case legs of the
dining table. I said that the food probably tasted just as good, to
which—'It's O.K. now that Mother's here!' There was a long pause
in the conversation and she remarked that she ought to have my
telephone number.

"Mother was timing the feed with her watch off her wrist.
When she took the nipple out of Charles's mouth and put him over
her left shoulder the watch dropped off her lap and I picked it up
for her. She patted his back firmly but not too hard, and he brought
up wind almost at once. He straightway began to shout and roar in
ever-increasing tones of anger, was not quietened by his mother's
talking to him, and when she gave him the right breast he made
several attempts to take the nipple, making a kissing sound as he
did so. The mother finally put the nipple right into his mouth and
he began to suck. This time I could see a bit better and he seemed
to be sucking very gently and slowly. There was the same motionless quality to his whole body as he sucked.

"As he began to suck he gave the breast a pat with his right
hand just above the nipple. His hand seemed to interfere with his
mouth (as it were, falling on to the nipple), so that the mother twice
moved his hand away. He finally arranged it in a trumpet shape
around his mouth. His feet were motionless, except that I noticed
he once made a small stroking action against the chair with one
foot. Mother said: 'Come on, work', very gently, and in a somewhat
resigned sort of way.

"After a certain time mother took Charles off the breast, very
sleepy, and first held him sitting up facing her, saying that Spock
advised winding this way before trying the shoulder method, but

that she had never had any luck with this nor heard of anyone who had. I agreed, and mentioned my own son and our experiences in winding him. She asked how old he was and remarked that Jack, Charles's brother, was 19 months old.

"The mother then put Charles over her shoulder, very sleepy and lolling and with a replete air. I don't recall that he brought up wind.

"She then put him back to the right breast, where he sucked even more slowly for a while. She then carried Charles against her shoulder upstairs to change him. I walked behind, and at this point Charles's face was quite calm but rather bloated and expressionless really. He was more in a stupor than asleep, it seemed, and made no sound.

"We went into the little room where the mother slept with Charles. The bed was unmade, and there was an empty chocolate wrapper beside it. The mother arranged the blanket on the bed and laid Charles on his back, at which he woke up quickly and began to scream. She left the room to fetch clean napkins. He continued to scream, both hands constantly round his face with pushing and scraping-off movements, his feet doing the same; pushing the left against and down the right.

"The screaming stopped when the mother called from another room, and was replaced for a moment by a happy low cooing sound. Then screams till the mother came back and talked sympathetically while she changed him. During the changing he cried miserably, but without drowning the sound of his mother's voice. His hands were constantly around his face, his left hand moving in front of him with a stroking action which reminded me of a blind man.

"The mother powdered his genitals and stomach generously, drew attention to his rash, and remarked that lots of babies around had such a rash. When he was changed, she laid him on his left side in the cot, leaving his hands free of the blanket which wrapped him. She then left to get Jack up from his sleep, as they were going for a walk.

"Charles lay with his left thumb in his mouth, the fingers of his left hand over his face, especially over the right eye (the left eye was turned somewhat into the sheet); his right hand was curling over his temple. He breathed fast and noisily, and irregularly from time to time. Then his left hand assumed the trumpet shape that his right hand had done during the feed. His face showed scarcely any movement. All at once there was a sudden, heavy, heaving sigh and he seemed to relax altogether. His breathing became inaudible, his hands moved slightly away from his face. Over the next few minutes he gave several jerks forward, his arms outstretched as though he was falling and clutching at someone. This seemed to happen sometimes to external stimuli. (The mother's voice talking to Jack in the next room, a door banging, and sometimes without any external stimulus that I noted.)

"Finally he lay quietly asleep. Two or three times he half woke at some loud noises from Jack's room, began to pucker and cry, but then fell asleep again. He began to cry when his mother came and put a cardigan and bonnet on him, treating him sympathetically and talking to him. He fell asleep again and was carried downstairs on the cot mattress which was going in the pram. As he lay on the mattress while the mother and grandmother gathered together things for the walk, I was struck by his expression, which had quite altered in the meantime and was now fixed in a look of great pain of an intense kind, and not a muscle moved for the two or three minutes between when I first saw it and when I said goodbye to them outside the house."

I have given this material in considerable detail to show the observer at work and the impact that this experience makes on him. Further, I want this baby to become familiar because I shall discuss other material from him later in this paper.

If we consider this material from the point of view of how it affected the observer, we naturally take into account that this was his first meeting with the family. The observer noted the mother's anxiety about how to deal with him. Between the lines the observer's tension can be discerned. He notes that the mother changes places with him so that grandmother in the garden can see the feed while he cannot. His sensitivity is registered in the record by calling the mother's invitation "muttered", and perhaps by misunderstanding her remark about times in the sense that she did not want him to see the feed. When, to the mother's apologies for the state of the house, particularly the dining table, he remarks that the food probably tastes just as good, the mother says it's O.K. now that her own mother is here. Here we can see the first glimpse of the mother's depression and dependence on her own mother and the observer's attempt at comforting her. "There was a long pause in the conversation and the mother remarked could she have my telephone number." That two relationships are going on—baby–breast, mother–observer—in relative isolation is evident. The observer's sympathy for the mother's depression comes through again when, after prolonged attempts at the second breast, the mother said to Charles, "Come on, work", and the observer notes she said it "gently, in a somewhat resigned sort of way".

Identification with the baby's misery (the scratched face) and later feeling of desertion in favour of the older brother whom the mother now went to awaken is written in each subsequent line. The mystery of the face scratches begins to be solved as both hands constantly move round his face with pushing and scraping-off movements, his feet doing the same, while the mother is out of the room.

After being changed the baby is seen to fall asleep, an event described by the observer vividly with great attention to detail, but on parting he was struck by Charles's expression, which had quite altered into a look of great pain of an intense kind although the baby was asleep. That the observer could have noted and reported in great detail with these tensions going on and in his first baby observation is striking.

The problem in such a paper as this is to convey the use that the seminar makes of such observations, and this I can do only to a very limited extent. To convey it correctly one would need to report the discussion in the seminar in as much detail as the observational material itself. And even this could give a fallacious impression since the deductions drawn necessarily depend upon previous observations and discussions, from which, slowly, series of observations can be linked and patterns of behaviour seen to emerge. The point that I am stressing here is the importance of consecutive observation of the individual couple. The experience of the seminar is that one may see an apparent pattern emerging in one observation, but one can only accept it as significant if it is repeated in the same, or a similar, situation in many subsequent observations. Paying attention to such observable details over a long period gives the student the opportunity to see not only patterns but also changes in the patterns. He can see changes in the couple's mutual adaptation and the impressive capacity for growth and development in their relationship, i.e. the flexibility and capacity for using each other and developing which goes on in a satisfactory mother–baby relationship. The excitement in the seminar has been just as much in searching backward as in looking forward.

I will give two examples of such patterns of behaviour from the same baby, Charles.

In the first observation the observer described the baby's difficulties when feeding at the second breast; how the feeding was slow, long drawn out, and how the mother remarked that he did not work hard—but went on with the feed. In later observations we began to see that this was part of a pattern in which he related himself differently to the two breasts. At the first breast he sucked vigorously, sometimes gulping, while at the second breast he sucked very gently, his mouth barely moving. The mother remarked on one occasion that he usually takes his meal at the first breast and "fiddles around", as she puts it, on the second. However, she persevered, taking him off and putting him back, saying that he would not sleep the right length of time if he did not get enough. At the second breast Charles also made many movements with his hands, patting, making the trumpet shape, holding to his mother's jersey, stroking.

Thus after some weeks we had noted the pattern in the way Charles related himself to the two breasts, but it was only later with additional material about the hand movements that certain links suggested themselves—and these I am going to discuss later.

Another pattern emerged from the second observation when the bathing was watched. Charles began to cry as soon as his napkins were taken off, but his crying became much more intense when his nightdress came off. It became fainter when his mother handled him, washed, soaped him and spoke to him softly. When put down on a sheet his crying became louder. Once back in his nightdress the crying stopped immediately; he relaxed and began to look around. This pattern of crying intensely when his body was exposed during the bath or when put down was repeated in every observation until the end of the second month. He was soothed by his mother's voice and her handling, but quietened immediately when wrapped up, i.e. in his nightdress, or covered with a blanket in the cot.

While the foregoing patterns seem to suggest the working of intrapsychic defensive operations, patterns of communication between mother and child can also be observed, in which the mother's fundamental role of "holding" in Winnicott's sense or containing projections in Bion's sense can be observed.

It becomes apparent that between a particular mother and child certain preferred modes of communication become central in their relation to one another. It is difficult to tell whether this choice originates in the mother's or the baby's preference. I would like to give two examples.

One of the mothers, whom I will call Mrs A., was uneasy in the feeding situation. She held the baby very awkwardly, and seemed tense and anxious at having the baby so close to her body. This is similar to the mother on whom I reported at the beginning of this paper, who also could not stand the close physical contact with the infant. Mrs A. showed that she was happiest when, after the feed was over, she would either put the baby comfortably on the floor or hold it with both arms away from her body. She would look at it, make movements with her lips (open and shut her mouth), to which the baby responded in the same way, or she would talk to the baby and the baby make various sounds back. One day, when the baby was in his fifth month, the mother had to go out shopping and left him with the observer to whom she gave various instructions. The observer sat down with the baby, and as long as he held it on his knee with its back to him, the baby was quiet. As soon as he started talking to the baby, or turned it round so that it could see him, it began to cry. This happened several times. In the discussion in the seminar it was felt that to this baby the association to a happy relation with mother was predominantly visual and vocal. The voice and sight of the observer was different from that of the mother, and awareness of this made the baby cry. It occurred to the observer that while the baby was sitting quietly on his knee it looked fixedly at the part of the room where the mother had been just before she left, as if it found comfort in looking at the area

which was connected with the mother, while the voice and sight of
the observer was proof that the mother was not there, and the baby
cried.

Here is a contrasting example in which the kinaesthetic pattern
is the key to the nature of the relationship. The observation began
when baby James was four and a half weeks old. His mother had
been undressing him in preparation for the bath. As she first put
him on his back he tried to reach for the breast and made some
protesting noises. The mother talked to him continually, saying,
"It's horrible, isn't it?" . . . "Poor old fellow, never mind, you will
soon be in the water." She told the observer that he loved actually
being in the water, unlike her other children who disliked it when
they were babies. When in the water he lay quietly bringing his
knees up to his stomach, making no sound and looking quite contented. In later observations he splashed, kicked, and played in the
bath and often protested when taken out, as at this first observation
when he was four and a half weeks old. Then when mother put him
on to the breast he attached himself to the nipple at once and
sucked vigorously. He had his eyes open and with the right hand
he touched the breast and the button on the mother's dress alternately. This touching of the mother's body was observed as a regular pattern of behaviour whenever the baby came close to her. At
thirteen weeks, the mother gave the observer the baby to hold
while she went out to prepare the bath and said, "Go to your
auntie, she's got to study you." James lay on the observer's lap
looking at her, but did not touch her. When the mother returned he
looked at her and followed her with his eyes until she took him. On
her lap he felt for the breast with mouth and hand and later held
her arm with his hand. After the bath, at the breast, he clutched at
the breast; his mother removed his hand. He then put his hand on
top of the mother's hand and moved it rhythmically while he
sucked. At twenty-two weeks he was stroking the breast with wide
movements. "At twenty-four weeks" (I am quoting from the student's notes) "James took the breast eagerly. His mother said he
would not be having it much longer, the milk was giving out. With
his left hand James played with the mother's breast and then with
her hand. His movements remained lively all through the taking of
the breast. As I watched him I wondered if his movements might

be a conscious caressing of the mother; he appeared to me to be aware of what his hand was doing. The mother put James to the second breast and he took this eagerly, stroking her breast and neck and touching her mouth, although usually I have only noticed him do this during the first breast. He was weaned to the bottle at twenty-seven weeks. There followed a week of distress when he refused food, falling asleep between mouthfuls, while sleeping badly at night. The mother remarked that he behaved as though he was a little baby. In the following week he started touching the bottle, later reaching out for it, stroking it lovingly, as he had done with the breast and eventually settled down to keeping one hand on the bottle and touching, stroking, and caressing the mother with the other hand."

I have, of course, described the overall patterns—the gross trends—and have had to omit the many finer details of the ups and downs, as time would not permit of recounting them. The material convinced us in the seminar that the relation of this baby to the breast and mother was close and intimate, and he expressed his love as well as anger towards her, predominantly by handling her body. We noted that although the mother was very vocal herself, the baby remained relatively silent, with a preference for tactile and kinaesthetic modes of relationship and communication.

Before closing I would like to mention some aspects of the baby observation as training for scientific data collection and thought. In the seminars it comes out very clearly from the beginning how difficult it is to "observe", i.e. collect facts free from interpretation. As soon as these facts have to be described in language we find that every word is loaded with a penumbra of implication. Should the student say the nipple "dropped" from the baby's mouth, "fell", was "pushed", "released", "escaped", etc.? In fact, he finds that he chooses a particular word because observing and thinking are almost inseparable. This is an important lesson, for it teaches caution and reliance on consecutive observations for confirmation.

What we also find is that the students learn to watch and feel before jumping in with theories, and learn to tolerate and appreciate how mothers care for their babies, and find their own solutions. In this way the students are slowly able to discard rather fixed notions about right and wrong handling and become more flexible

about accepted principles of infant care. What is borne in upon
them is the uniqueness of each couple, how each baby develops at
its own pace and relates itself to its mother in its own way.

Probably the most exciting aspect of the seminars, as they
develop during the year, is the opportunity for teasing out of
the material certain threads of behaviour which seem particularly
significant for a particular child's experience of his own object
relations. An item may strike the group as having a meaningful
configuration. Its earlier history can then be traced in the notes,
hypotheses made and predictions evolved for validation in further
observations. For instance, it will be remembered that in the first
observation with baby Charles, at ten days, it was noted that he
patted the second, right breast and formed a trumpet shape with
his hand around his mouth as he sucked away very gently and
slowly. When left alone on the bed later his right hand was exploring around his eye and temple while his left thumb was in his
mouth. Then gradually his left hand assumed the trumpet shape
and all at once he went to sleep.

The fact that hand activity was an important mode of contact
with his object and his body seemed clear in a general way, but of
no special interest until the observations at 9 and 10 weeks. The
observer reports: 9 weeks—after a disturbed feed because of a
change in routine, Charles played with his hands in a complex
way. First one hand seemed to be plucking and squeezing the
other, twisting the fingers and thumb quite hard. Occasionally one
hand described a small circle in front of his mouth while his face
had a disagreeable, discontented expression, rather screwed up.
After this a change came about. He became very much calmer and
played with his hands in a much more playful way bringing them
together, rubbing them and poking his fingers through each other.
Put to the right breast he sucked regularly. His hands were on each
side of the breast well away from the nipple The mother remarked
that he often touched the breast while feeding with a pat and a
poke, quite hard.

"10 weeks—his mother had her hand on his chest and he began
to play with her fingers, curling his own round hers and gently
drawing his forefinger along her wrist and hand. He also looked at
her face and made friendly sounds in response to her talk. Prior to
this, at the left (first) breast where he sucked powerfully and regu-

larly, his right hand was lying high up in the centre of the mother's chest. Then he began to stop and resume sucking. During the stopping his right hand began to clutch and clench markedly. Later at the right breast he sucked less regularly. He had both hands on the breast close to the nipple on each side and gently moved his fingers on the breast, occasionally bringing his hands momentarily together.

"From now onwards a definite pattern could be observed. When he was at the right (second) breast he would stroke and caress the breast in a variety of gentle movements, but when he was at the left breast his hand was either on the mother's chest, his fingers sometimes clenching, or both hands were on either side of the breast, motionless.

"We were struck by the way in which the hands related to each other, at first twisting, plucking, squeezing rather hard, later rubbing and poking the fingers through each other playfully. At the next observation Charles was seen to play in this second way with the mother's hand after the feed at the first breast, at which he had alternated between powerful sucking and stopping, while his right hand clenched and unclenched when his mouth was inactive. We could see in the seminar a strong suggestion here of his hand being mouthlike in its activities and mother's hand being breastlike in its significance, thus suggesting that his two hands might at times also be relating to each other as mouth to breast.

"When put to the second breast Charles sucked gently, having both his hands on the breast near the nipple, gently caressing and occasionally bringing his hands together. In contrast, at the first breast powerful sucking alternated with hand clenching, the hand being held far away from the nipple."

As I have indicated earlier in this paper, this split in his relation to the two breasts and the accompanying pattern of hand activity subsequently became quite firmly established. Whichever way we may attempt to explain it, the vital significance of these minute activities is undeniable. Charles clearly relates himself to the two breasts in a very different way. His hand tends to behave like a mouth. He brings his hands close to the second breast but away from the first. He treats his mother's hand with his hand as his mouth treats the breast. His hands relate to each other at times as mouth to breast just as his mouth relates to his hand as a breast. Is this evidence that the relationship to the breast as part-object is the basic unit of relationship from which more complex relationships are built? Is the poking through and the poking in of fingers evidence of a projective mode of achieving identification? Are the hands held away and the clenching alternating with powerful sucking to be seen as a primitive attempt to spare the breast? Innumerable exciting questions arise, showing the students the vast area of the unconscious still to be explored by psycho-analysis.

My impression is that the students find the observational evidence for the early working of the splitting processes and identification of body parts with objects fascinating, regardless of the theoretical framework within which they may choose to express the recognition of infant mental functioning. I think that the infant observation experience, linked later with clinical experience with adults and children, will add to their conviction of the importance of observing patients' overall behaviour as a part of the data of the analytic situation as well as strengthen their belief in the validity of analytic reconstruction of early development.

CHAPTER THREE

The experience of the skin
in early object relations

[1968]

The central theme of this brief communication is concerned with the primal function of the skin of the baby and of its primal objects in relation to the most primitive binding together of parts of the personality not as yet differentiated from parts of the body. It can be most readily studied in psychoanalysis in relation to problems of dependence and separation in the transference.

The thesis is that in its most primitive form the parts of the personality are felt to have no binding force among themselves and must therefore be held together in a way that is experienced by them passively, by the skin functioning as a boundary. But this internal function of containing the parts of the self is dependent initially on the introjection of an external object, experienced as capable of fulfilling this function. Later, identification with this function of the object supersedes the unintegrated state and gives

---

Read at the 25th International Psycho-Analytical Congress, Copenhagen, July 1967.

rise to the fantasy of internal and external spaces. Only then the stage is set for the operation of primal splitting and idealization of self and object as described by Melanie Klein. Until the containing functions have been introjected, the concept of a space within the self cannot arise. Introjection, i.e. construction of an object in an internal space is therefore impaired. In its absence, the function of projective identification will necessarily continue unabated and all the confusions of identity attending it will be manifest.

The stage of primal splitting and idealization of self and object can now be seen to rest on this earlier process of containment of self and object by their respective "skins".

The fluctuations in this primal state will be illustrated in case material, from infant observation, in order to show the difference between unintegration as a passive experience of total helplessness, and disintegration through splitting processes as an active defensive operation in the service of development. We are, therefore, from the economic point of view, dealing with situations conducive to catastrophic anxieties in the unintegrated state as compared with the more limited and specific persecutory and depressive ones.

The need for a containing object would seem, in the infantile unintegrated state, to produce a frantic search for an object—a light, a voice, a smell, or other sensual object—which can hold the attention and thereby be experienced, momentarily at least, as holding the parts of the personality together. The optimal object is the nipple in the mouth, together with the holding and talking and familiar smelling mother.

Material will show how this containing object is experienced concretely as a skin. Faulty development of this primal skin function can be seen to result either from defects in the adequacy of the actual object or from fantasy attacks on it, which impair introjection. Disturbance in the primal skin function can lead to a development of a "second-skin" formation through which dependence on the object is replaced by a pseudo-independence, by the inappropriate use of certain mental functions, or perhaps innate talents, for the purpose of creating a substitute for this skin container function. The material to follow will give some examples of "second-skin" formation.

Here I can only indicate the types of clinical material upon which these findings are based. My present aim is to open up this topic for a detailed discussion in a later paper.

Infant observation: Baby Alice

One year of observation of an immature young mother and her first baby showed a gradual improvement in the "skin-container" function up to twelve weeks. As the mother's tolerance to closeness to the baby increased, so did her need to excite the baby to manifestations of vitality lessen. A consequent diminution of unintegrated states in the baby could be observed. These had been characterized by trembling, sneezing, and disorganized movements. There followed a move to a new house in a still unfinished condition. This disturbed severely the mother's holding capacity and led her to a withdrawal from the baby. She began feeding while watching television, or at night in the dark without holding the baby. This brought a flood of somatic disturbance and an increase of unintegrated states in the baby. Father's illness at that time made matters worse and the mother had to plan to return to work. She began to press the baby into a pseudo-independence, forcing her onto a training-cup, introducing a bouncer during the day, while harshly refusing to respond to the crying at night. The mother now returned to an earlier tendency to stimulate the child to aggressive displays which she provoked and admired. The result by six and a half months was a hyperactive and aggressive little girl, whom her mother called "a boxer" from her habit of pummelling people's faces. We see here the formation of a muscular type of self-containment—"second-skin" in place of a proper skin container.

Analysis of a schizophrenic girl: Mary

Some years of analysis, since age 3½, have enabled us to reconstruct the mental states reflected in the history of her infantile disturbance. The facts are as follows: a difficult birth, early clenching of the nipple but lazy feeding, bottle supplement in the third week but on breast until 11 months, infantile eczema at 4 months and scratching until bleeding, extreme clinging to mother, severe intolerance to waiting for feeds, delayed and atypical development in all areas.

In the analysis, severe intolerance to separation was reflected from the start as in the jaw-clenched systematic tearing and breaking of all materials after the first holiday-break. Utter dependence on the immediate contact could be seen and studied in the unintegrated states of posture and motility on the one hand, and thought and communication on the other, which existed at the beginning of each session, improving during the course, to reappear on leaving. She came in hunched, stiff-jointed, grotesque like a "sack of potatoes" as she later called herself, and emitting an explosive "SSBICK" for "Good morning, Mrs Bick". This "sack of potatoes" seemed in constant danger of spilling out its contents partly due to the continual picking of holes in her skin representing the "sack" skin of the object in which parts of herself, the "potatoes", were contained (projective identification). Improvement from the hunched posture to an erect one was achieved, along with a lessening of her general total dependence, more through a formation of a second skin based on her own muscularity than on identification with a containing object.

Analysis of an adult neurotic patient

The alternation of two types of experience of self—the "sack of apples" and "the hippopotamus"—could be studied in regard to quality of contact in the transference and experience of separation, both being related to a disturbed feeding period. In the "sack of apples" state, the patient was touchy, vain, in need of constant attention and praise, easily bruised and constantly expecting catastrophe, such as a collapse when getting up from the couch. In the "hippopotamus" state, the patient was aggressive, tyrannical, scathing, and relentless in following his own way. Both states were related to the "second-skin" type of organization, dominated by projective identification. The "hippopotamus" skin, like the "sack", were a reflection of the object's skin inside which he existed, while the thin-skinned, easily bruised, apples inside the sack represented that state of parts of the self which were inside this insensitive object.

Analysis of a child: Jill

Early in the analysis of a 5-year-old child, whose feeding period had been characterized by anorexia, skin-container problems presented themselves, as in her constant demand from mother during the first analytic holiday, that her clothes should be firmly fastened, her shoes tightly laced. Later material showed her intense anxiety and need to distinguish herself from toys and dolls, about which she said: "Toys are not like me, they break to pieces and don't get well. They don't have a skin. We have a skin!"

Summary

In all patients with disturbed first-skin formation, severe disturbance of the feeding period is indicated by analytic reconstruction, though not always observed by the parents. This faulty skin-formation produces a general fragility in later integration and organizations. It manifests itself in states of unintegration as distinct from regression involving the most basic types of partial or total unintegration of body, posture, motility, and corresponding functions of mind, particularly communication. The "second-skin" phenomenon which replaces first skin integration, manifests itself as either partial or total type of muscular shell or a corresponding verbal muscularity.

Analytic investigation of the second skin phenomenon tends to produce transitory states of unintegration. Only an analysis which perseveres to thorough working-through of the primal dependence on the maternal object can strengthen this underlying fragility. It must be stressed that the containing aspect of the analytic situation resides especially in the setting and is therefore an area where firmness of technique is crucial.

CHAPTER FOUR

Further considerations on the function of the skin in early object relations

Findings from infant observation
integrated into child and adult analysis

[1986]

In 1968 I presented a paper built around clinical experiences and infant observations "concerned with the primal function of the skin of the baby and of its primal objects in relation to the most primitive binding together of parts of the personality not as yet differentiated from parts of the body" (Bick, 1968). There I described some of the evidence suggesting that in the earliest times the parts of the personality are felt to have no inherent binding force and fall apart unless passively held together, an experience indistinguishable from feeling the body to be held together by the skin. The suggestion was also made that in the event of defective development of this containment function other "secondary skin" devices may arise, in collaboration with particularities of the maternal care, such as muscular or vocal methods. The consequences for personality development were briefly illustrated, with special reference to ego strength, pseudo-independence and tendency to disintegration.

In the present communication I wish to extend those findings and to investigate them in greater depth. The same child, Mary, whose material served originally, will most usefully open the area to investigation if described in somewhat greater detail. She came to me for analysis at the age of three and a half years for reasons of severe general retardation which relentlessly followed on from a difficult birth; the mother had a Caesarean section after a pro-longed and futile attempt to deliver her normally. In the very first week she manifested severe clamping on the nipple so that it could hardly be removed from her mouth, and in the second week the mother lost much of her milk. Mary then became a lazy feeder but was always impatient to come to the breast, which she would not surrender until she was eleven months old. She was quite intoler-ant to separation from the outset, so that mother could never go out in the evenings, all of which was greatly aggravated when she developed eczema at four and a half months of age. Her night-time scratching was so severe, to the point of bleeding, that she had to sleep with her mother, who held her hands as the only method of both restraining and calming her.

At the beginning of analysis her retardation in speech, toilet habits and motor control was severe. She needed her mother to put her on the pot, to wipe her usually streaming nose, to fasten her shoelaces; she was "spilling out" as she later told me. But the first three months brought a most encouraging change in general liveli-ness, speech and emotional contact. Her parents told me she could not wait to come to me and that she called me Bicki or Choki Biki. When it was time to go she could not get up and made efforts to tear herself away as if she were stuck to the chair. Later in the analysis she told me that she would spill out should she get up. When she eventually got to the door, she would hold on to the knob with one hand, turned it round and round, then at last opened the door, banged it, then smiling said "good-bye". This seemed to me to repeat the impatience to come to the nipple and to hold on to it with such strength that according to mother and nurses she stretched it to one and a half inches before she let it go.

She often repeated phrases from my interpretations, such as "I think it's a man like daddy", and I tended to assume that she was employing projective identification to lose herself in identification with me. But the first break at Christmas produced a dramatic change which forced me to alter my ideas and puzzle over the multitude of phenomena she now exhibited. On her return she started a systematic destruction of the play materials, teeth clenched, stopping only to pick up bits in order to tear them or break them into smaller bits. I was reminded of the history of her relentless scratching and tearing of the skin until she bled—spilled out. This behaviour changed when she indicated I should pick up all the bits when she threw them in my direction. Gradually the destruction was replaced by a ball game in which she had complete control over my movements. I had to stay in a certain place and was only allowed to hold the ball to my chest when she threw it to me; she then took it back and went into a position opposite me and threw the ball again. This process was repeated until we neared the end of the session when it would be replaced by her spinning a tin, excitedly flapping her hands as she watched. It seems that she repeated bodily in her flapping the movement and rhythm of the spinning tin.

It was then that I began to wonder about the nature of the identification that produced the parroting of my phrases, and realized that I was seeing a very complicated process in fragmented form repeating her developmental history. I construed that the tin was the nipple to which she was stuck as by a centrifugal force and could not let go—as she was stuck to the chair, her hand to the doorknob—as she needed to be held by mother's hands, by her continuous presence. Being separated meant being torn away and torn to pieces by persecuting hands, like the ones that destroyed the play material and had earlier scratched her skin to bleeding. The desperate clinging for survival was mounted in the face of an experience of lacerating separation which would let her life leak away like a liquid substance. It therefore seemed likely that the identification and consequent mimicry of my phrases was due to her sticking on to my surface, and I came to think of it as an adhesive identification rather than a projective one.

Somewhat later I learned more about the difficulty of disengaging a relationship of the adhesive sort through supervising the treatment of Sonia, aged six and a half. It was carried out by a sensitive young man who carried the maternal transference well for her. This child, the youngest of three, had been born after a prolonged labour and was breastfed for four months. At fifteen months she had convulsions during febrile chicken pox, and at twenty months a cancer of the retina required removal of the eye, so that she now wears a glass eye. The possibility of an epilectic tendency was realized at four years and controlled by phenobarbitone. By the time of referral she manifested a disturbed general development. The parents reported that she repeatedly ran out of the house, had no sense of danger and that she had a fantasy twin called Rosy. At school she was always running to the headmaster, to the caretaker or to one particular odd boy. They found her ineducable. Sonia's mother suffered from depression and had to be hospitalized at times. Her father's relationship to her seemed to be of the adhesive kind, as observed by the therapist. In the waiting-room she had to sit close to the father and when she went with the therapist he followed her with his eyes a long way and waved. He objected to the treatment and insisted on controlling its length. The therapist had to negotiate for the continuity at half-yearly intervals. It seems that Sonia's running to the two caretaking men at school was determined by her need to cling to father figures while the odd boy was probably felt by her to be the twin Rosy—the "same" as she. Later in the analysis when she became concerned about having one eye she expressed the urgent desire to go to live with an uncle who like herself had only one eye.

Before the weekend of her analysis Sonia started very interesting separation rituals. She drew first two joining loops and then a long row of them. She spoke of her twin who would stay with her over the weekend. When she came back on Monday she proceeded to move following the pattern of the row of loops. With the right hand she held the door-knob, with the left the wall next to her. She walked over the furniture of the room not touching the ground and looping to the wall. When she came to the highest point at the end of the furniture she scraped the plaster from the ceiling, pointed to the dust that covered the floor and said "That is to stop the gap." The looping to the wall on Monday was a reunion ritual.

For Sonia the wall seemed to be a concrete representation of her mother's body to which she could hold. The sink with the water was also used for a separation ritual and could be seen to represent her mother's lap and nipple. Her last move at the end of each session was to go to the sink. There she lay on the sink, put her mouth round the tap and filled her mouth with water. She held the water until her mother came into sight as she approached the waiting-room, whereupon she swallowed the water and held on to the mother with her eyes. The number of mouthfuls she took was proportioned to the duration of separation before weekends and holidays. There was also a phenomenon of turning cartwheels in which she was very skilful, and very ritualized skipping games with which she usually ended the session. I think that these were attempts at muscular hyperkinetic self-containment—second skin formation—when she stood before the gap.

Before the first holiday the ritual was augmented by drawing a letter J for Jew. She said that Jewish children had double holidays. She did not stop her line however at the end of the letter J, but calling it "the dead-end" she appeared very anxious. She continued the line in parallel to the letter round and round. I concluded that Sonia found the existence of the gap—falling to death—threatening, just as the looping was an expression of twinning and similar to the way she attached herself to any available person. She had similarly noticed that Jewish children were not "the same as the others", just as she was not the same "because of the glass eye". She too had double holidays, from school and from analysis.

I began to think of adhesive identification as a defence against the dead-end, but it was only when I began to think of the adhesive identification and the dead-end together in relation to dimensionality that I came to see how it was different from other persecutory fears.

An adult patient Mrs B. helped me to see this more clearly, for she brought into the analysis extreme difficulties with listening and thinking. She regularly wept "buckets" in the Thursday session. One Thursday she told me that the worst thing in the world must be to be told you have a "terminal disease". Friday was her "terminal disease", and listening on Thursday would have brought her this information and the necessity to think about it. Her world was two-dimensional, a so-called "flat earth" for whom the dead-end meant falling into space. Another patient Mrs S. showed a similar relation to the unknown. To be without an answer was like "sinking into the quicksand". On a Thursday she brought a dream: five little lambs seemed to be in the consulting-room with us and the fourth lamb said crying to the fifth that on Friday he would have to die. But if he listened to the analyst reading a book he would survive. The implication is that on Friday she would be able to survive the weekend gap in her knowledge of my life by covering that gap with information gleaned from listening very carefully and from watching. For instance by making a link between there being irises in my hall and hearing a colleague who had irises in her garden speak in praise of my work she could construe that I spent my weekends with that person. The hole in her knowledge was closed. She would not fall into the quicksand of bottomless dead-end.

From patients such as Mrs B. and Mrs S. I began to see that an adhesive relationship was on-the-surface of the object and two-dimensional, while every separation and discontinuity (in knowledge of the object, for instance) was the unknown third dimension, the fall into space. It was interesting to hear from Mrs A. that as a child her father had extreme difficulty putting her to sleep for, although reading to her induced slumber, the moment his hands touched the door-knob to leave her little eyes popped open again. How like Mary with the nipple, Sonia with the water held in her mouth. This realization of the falling-through-space aspect of the dead-end took me back to experiences of observing mother–infant interaction. There I could begin to see evidence of the genesis of these difficulties in detail, so that vague formulations referable, say, to maternal depression could be replaced by more precise insight.

I will now bring an example from an infant observation. In fact infant observation is a misnomer because the observer is observing the family to whom an infant has been born. From material over many years one can see that the fundamental problem for each member of the family is the change of identity experienced in various degrees. The mother feels she has lost her identity as a capable adult in control of her time and activities. Instead she is assailed from all sides by overwhelming demands: the demand to be a perfect mother, to have nothing for herself, not even sleep. These feelings have their roots in her own infantile complaints about the inadequacy of her own mother.

The older child who has a staple identity as mummy's baby is dispossessed; he no longer knows who he is and often regresses to the level of a baby and becomes distracted and fights for his survival. All this increases mother's guilt. Some mothers are driven to stop breast-feeding as they cannot bear the suffering of the older child. The father can be a great support at this time if he can take over the mothering, but often he too feels dispossessed and displaced.

In many cases an observer can help when he can stay in his role of sympathetic listener because all that mother wants is to unburden herself. Advice means a further demand on her. An observer in a family with a new baby is exposed to intense feelings and is often drawn into identification particularly with the suffering of the baby, so that he feels critical of the mother. For instance I have noticed two striking situations where the observer feels particularly upset. One is when the mother takes the baby away from the nipple to wind him and does it very frequently; the other is when she is bathing the baby. She herself seems terrified that she will let the baby fall.

I had an opportunity to discuss this with a professor of paediatrics who told me that bathing is not really essential at such an early stage and mother could just wash him. But with regard to the wind there is a problem of adaptation after birth because he explained that *in utero* there is no sense of gravity. When the baby is born he is in the position of an astronaut who has been shot out into outer space without a spacesuit.

Here is an example from an observation on a three-week-old baby seen by an intuitive observer. I quote:

> Before the baby brought up his wind his face, body and hands seemed to open and close, his body bunched and unbunched, his face screwed up and relaxed. Mother then laid him on her lap so that his feet were pointing to her stomach. When put down his hands and feet flew out almost like an astronaut in a gravity-less zone. She responded by talking gently to him again and bringing both his hands down to his stomach with her hands. She then laid him on the changing pad saying that he did not usually like to be changed.

Through this identification with the baby the observer can intuit that the predominant terror of the baby is of falling to pieces or liquefying. One can see this in the infant trembling and quivering when the nipple is taken out of his mouth, but also when his clothes are taken off.

Here is an example from an infant observation. This is the first baby of a young couple. When the observer came to arrange the times, before the baby was born, the mother was preoccupied with her need for a new dress. She would have to have it for Christmas parties or she would be unfit to be seen. This was the first sign of her fear of identity: "unfit to be seen". Next she said that baby must sit up soon and she had seen a chair and was going to buy it for the baby. She was also afraid of her parents coming lest the baby be deformed or dead. She would be blamed for it. She doubted whether her husband would be there at the birth, because he thought that messy, and he did not like messy children. In fact this father felt very much excluded and the weekends were particularly distressing. Mother felt persecuted by the baby and so did father, for the baby "did not leave them alone"; when he cried before dinner father would say "Oh no, I am not going to eat alone again."

The example of the chair for the baby was indicating mother's feeling that she was not able to provide a lap for the baby to sit on. Mother's eagerness for a chair was a harbinger of a most distressing feature. In fact she could not hold the baby for any length of time and when she was feeding him the bottle she turned him away from herself. At the first observation at seventeen days, she immediately handed the baby to the observer asking whether the observer would nurse him—that is to say, be the chair. The observation of the baby in detail was extremely interesting though distressing, for he constantly moved his head from left to right, from right to left, also moving his hands, while the lower part of the body was quite immobile. At one point the baby managed to lift one hand, then the other hand to join the first one for support, and then both of them were lifted so that the fingers touched the face and held on to it. There were no further movements of the head. He was holding himself. When the mother then took him because he was apparently looking sleepy and she was hoping that she could now put him down, he grasped her hair and came quite near with his face to her neck. Mother was quite moved and murmured "You are cuddling me."

This indeed shows how strong his own need was to be held but also mother's need to be "cuddled—mothered". These integrated movements of this baby to touch his face seem to me a remarkable feat of organization in the service of survival. The mother usually left him—she told the observer—for about three hours lying alone and he only whimpered, but when he cried a bit louder she came up to him and just touched him and then he went to sleep for another hour. This baby had to make the most of his mother just touching him so that he could go to sleep again. During the bath when the mother took off the clothes he started quivering and shivering. One could perhaps suggest that he was cold because the clothes were taken off, but that was made unlikely by the fact that when mother touched him with a piece of wet cotton wool he also stopped shivering. I would suggest that this touching derives its power from its significance as an adhesion, as a re-establishment of feeling stuck on to mother.

This baby, like all other babies that we have observed, when not held by his mother clung at times in other ways. He would focus on a continuous sensory stimulus as for example a light or a continuous sound like that of the washing-machine. By holding on to it, be it with the eyes or with the ears as with the touch, the organs would serve as suction pads like a mouth holding on to the nipple. At this early stage there does not seem to be any differentiation of the separate functions; they all serve as suction pads for adhesion. The need to cling applies in a similar way to the mother. One mother who in order to protect her husband at night when the baby cried went to another room with the baby. She described what comfort it was to her to see the light from the Post Office Tower and to hear the hooting of an owl. She too was clinging in her distress with her eyes and ears to something sensual, different from the background, that she could focus on. This mother too has lost her spacesuit.

To go back to the baby: at three and a half months this baby's development seemed unsatisfactory in many ways that suggested a two dimensional relationship being enlarged only by addition of new features and not in complexity. For instance, he would invent a game of turning his head alternately to the mother and then to the observer as a way of holding their attention and even, with their encouragement, could extend this to imitating their sounds. But it was noticed that he could not take things to his mouth nor grasp them with his hands. For instance, when mother put him to sleep it was her habit to put a soft rabbit by his side. He would then manipulate the rabbit on to the *back* of his hands balancing it quite skilfully. But he did not grasp it.

Let me cite a contrasting example which also has a suggestive link to Sonia's loops and cartwheels. Baby B's mother seemed able to have a warm and sensitive relation to the child and it was noticed that he tended to make looping movements with his arms towards the breast when he was reunited with the mother at feeding times. He was bottle-fed and as the mother was right-handed the baby had only his left hand free. One day when he was sitting down mother put some toys near him on his left side. He began threshing with both arms, becoming more and more frantic. This pattern was noticed again and again whenever toys were put on his left side, but when they were placed to the right he made a perfect looping movement with his left arm and grasped them. It seemed very clear that this skill was connected with his looping movements towards the mother's breast during the bottle feed.

This example suggests how important the orientation towards the mother's body is for the baby to be able to grasp objects and explore them, namely that this capacity is founded on the primal relation to the grasping, clinging adhesive contact with the mother. Baby B had this relation towards the right and with his left hand, but when objects were on his left a state of disorganization and panic ensued. Baby A, in contrast, seemed to lack this grasping orientation. Adult patients in analysis can manifest similar difficulties in grasping ideas. Mrs S. surprised me and herself one day when she found a word of her own to describe her experience of herself instead of only being able to repeat my words. She said of herself: "I am a centipede, only in my country it is called a millipede". What surprised her most was that this new word came from "inside herself". In being able to recognize herself as a centipede, as a person whose only mode of adaptation was by holding on with a hundred hands, she had made a move   *towards* being a person with an inside where ideas could be found.

One Monday she brought the following dream: in it she had gone to visit a woman's house and found her with two children. They went to church together and her own two children seemed to be there as well. Then the woman told her to take all four children and leave. It was a weekend dream but what the four children meant I left for further elucidation. The number four kept on repeating in other dreams. Some time later, when I had the occasion to interpret some material as "sticking like a leech", she told me that when as a child she saw her father come into the house she would run and leap upon him, wrapping both her arms and legs around him and would refuse to be put down. We could then understand the dream, understand who the four children were.

This brings me to some comments regarding the technical problems related to analysis of patients with difficulties of the type I am trying to describe. These problems of ego strength, two-dimensionality, adhesive identification and second-skin formation lie very deep in the unconscious and have their origin early in the preverbal period. For these reasons, and because of the cata-strophic anxieties of the dead-end, falling through space, liquefy-ing, life-spilling-out variety attending them, they will not become available for analytic scrutiny *in the transference* unless the setting has been extremely constant and the technique extremely firm. Only when they feel well-contained in the transference will mate-rial begin to reflect the separation conflicts in ways that can be investigated with precision. Lacking this, splitting of the transfer-ence and acting out of the dependence in the face of separations defeat the investigation by aborting the emotionality. It is neces-sary to avoid too rapid formulations of well-known mechanisms, although they may be in evidence also, in favour of a more patient approach, waiting for repeated experiences to impress their pat-tern upon the patient.

As a result of work with such patients and the correlation with infant observations I began to see that another feature of the two-dimensionality and the clinging adhesive way of relating was the tendency to cling with eyes and ears as well as skin-to-skin and that this favoured a certain passivity, an observer rather than par-ticipant attitude towards life. This could be added then to the types of second-skin formation. An experience in Sonia's analysis later on threw a very bright light on the essentially unsatisfactory qual-ity of these second-skin attempts at self-containment. During an Easter holiday her mother had a depressive breakdown requiring hospital care and Sonia could only come three times per week to treatment for a while. The first time her mother was again able to take her, at the end of the session Sonia took firm hold of her therapist's thumb and led him to her mother in order to be able to ask, holding on to him, if her mother could bring her the next day again, as in former times. This holding of the thumb and being able to ask seemed a great move from holding water in her mouth and having to pass from therapist to mother without a gap. In fact her hand-looping and cart-wheeling had stopped and had been replaced by the construction of a tunnel leading from the couch to the tap of the sink. As she took her drink she explained that she was now a little baby who could get inside and no longer a stupid duck who thought it could fly by just flapping its wings. The cartwheels adhesive identification had given way to introjection and projective identification with an interval object.

Discussion and summary

Other workers have taken an interest in the infantile background of the processes that we have become accustomed to studying in analysis, those of projection and introjection, defensive operations, etc. Phyllis Greenacre has put forward interesting ideas about what she calls the "early ontogenetically appearing organismal defences and their transformation into the mental mechanisms of defence of the matured ego". Eugenio Gaddini has paid special attention to the role of the primitive imitation or mimicry in the formation of the processes of identification. In my own work I have tried to trace the processes of the most primitive holding together of the infantile body-ego, as they are fashioned jointly by mother-and-child-in-the-family, in order to demonstrate the steps necessary for the operation of projection, introjection and splitting and idealization.

Defects in this early containment of the personality may be devasting and obvious or subtle and covert depending on economic considerations. But I would suggest that where such impairment exists every new step in development is made more difficult and its outcome rendered more uncertain. The catastrophic anxiety of falling-into-space, the dead-end, haunts every demand for change and engenders a deep conservatism and demand for sameness, stability and support from the outside world. This may be masked where a second-skin formation is a prominent feature of character, but sudden collapse under stress reveals the flawed personality, well-adjusted as it may appear to be. In my experience, such patients in analysis require a slow firmly contained process with prolonged working through of each step forward in their development.

PART II

PUSHING AT THE BOUNDARIES

CHAPTER FIVE

Three years of observation with Mrs Bick

Jeanne Magagna

S ome years ago, in 1981, Mrs Martha Harris, Head of Child Psychotherapy Training, who was at that time the organizing tutor of the Tavistock Child Psychotherapy Course, contacted me to lead an infant observation seminar for social workers. Although I had observed one infant before, I felt inadequately equipped for the task, and so I asked Mrs Bick for supervision of my observation of a newly born baby. In 1948, when she began teaching at the Tavistock Clinic, she initiated the training method of having psychotherapy trainees visit a family and observe the development of an infant from birth to the age of 2 years. I am describing her method of infant observation in this chapter.

I began the observation of the infant and his family when Mrs Bick was 79 years old. This was her last formal teaching experience. Mrs Bick had at that time published three articles on the importance of infant observation, and she was intensely interested in pursuing the contribution of infant observation to psychoanalytic work. She was also very well known by former students as having

This is a modified version of a paper published in the *Journal of Child Psychotherapy*, 13 (No. 1, 1987).

extremely exacting standards for the observations. Mrs Bick was
eager to have every little detail of the observation, in order that she
should experience with Proustian clarity the relationship between
the baby and his family. I was aware that she was facing the end of
her life as the baby began his. It seemed to me that her own "in-
touchness" with the anxieties of dying enabled her to bring alive
with utmost sensitivity the baby's fears of dissolution. Mrs Bick
had such an enthusiasm for infant observation that somehow my
individual supervision with her became a seminar of six to thirteen
child psychotherapists who were doing a second infant observation. One year of observing became extended to three years of
weekly observations, which I presented to the seminar.

In this chapter, I examine areas of special difficulty in the beginning, middle, and last phases of this three-year observation. I shall
look at the following areas to illustrate some of Mrs Bick's central
ideas:

1.   the child in relation to his family;
2.   the role of the observer in containing the mother/baby anxie-
     ties;
3.   the role of the tutor and seminar members in helping the ob-
     server.

Initial stage—preparing for a new task

How do you prepare for a new task? Mrs Bick spent several seminars describing in detail how I should introduce myself to the
professional worker—in this case, a health visitor—who would
find a mother. She indicated a simple way of introducing baby
observation to the mother. I should say to the mother: "I want to
know more about babies and how they develop. I would find that
useful." The arrangement with the mother included meeting with
the father to acknowledge how my visits would affect both parents.
Also, my meeting the father indicated that I considered him to be
crucial for the baby's development. I was to introduce myself as
simply as possible as someone wanting more understanding of
babies, rather than as a professional, as a child psychotherapist.

I was to set a regular day, time, and hour limit of the visit as well as delineating possible times when I would not be visiting—Christmas, Easter, and August. There was to be a regular commitment to the specific times of meeting the family, just as there is in therapy arrangements with a patient. This was considered crucial to the task of the observations. Our seminar discussions about the visits stressed accommodating the mother so that she would feel that I was not making demands on her or intruding upon her desires for rest, her routine, or the baby's sleep. I was to be the psychologically containing person receptive to the family as much as possible, rather than someone requiring the family to be available to meet my needs. Making changes in appointments was considered to be making demands on the family and disrupting their routine. Being emotionally present for the family's sake was emphasized sufficiently for me to withstand the initial stresses of visiting.

The first observation: baby boy, 12 days old

The first visit after the birth was delayed, because the mother had had a Caesarian requiring over a week in hospital.

After my arrival, Mother, a tall, attractive, quiet-spoken lady in her late twenties, explains that the first two days at home have been terrible, but today, the day I visit, the baby was settled. They'd felt like two proud parents, going through the park with a new pram, a new baby. She adds, "we felt conspicuous and a bit silly because everything was so new". In a friendly way, the father—a highly educated, handsome, wealthy doctor in his late twenties—asks questions as to why I am coming, and he then gives a detailed account of the time before and after the baby's birth. He describes how four weeks before the birth everything was okay, but then the baby ended up in breach position. He adds that he argued with the doctor to see the delivery but he was not allowed to. When he saw the baby, his face was squashed. "It was a terrible mess." Father says that he is terribly worried that the baby might not be all right, might have difficulty feeding or talking because he has a very high palate. He adds that, because of the Caesarean and anaesthetic preventing Mother from seeing the baby, his wife felt that she was in hospital following an automobile accident, rather than because she was having a baby. Mother did not see the baby for the first two days in which the baby was in intensive care..

Meanwhile Mother is feeding the baby. When she sits him up to burp him, he raises his arms and gazes into the window, lifting his legs slightly. Back at the breast the baby's hands are clenched, while his arm rests along his side. His knees are drawn up and his toes slightly curled up. Mother's hand is wrapped around his leg, but baby isn't held very closely to her. Mother says the nurse told her to wrap the baby tightly in a blanket when feeding, but she didn't do this because she felt that some babies might like to move about and not feel cramped. Mother adds that she is anaemic, doesn't have much milk, and is worried that baby is getting too little. She has rented a scale to weigh him before and after feeds, to see if he is feeding. Mother supplements her milk with bottle-feeding at this point. While waiting for father to get the bottle, she burps the baby again. She then seats him on her knee and faces him outwards in my direction. He arches his neck with his head bent backwards so that his eyes look up in the direction of her face. She rubs his back, pats it slightly, and comments that babies arch their heads like that when they have wind.

Father returns with the bottle saying how he'd become an "old hand at it". He is worried about baby gulping down milk from the bottle. When Father later touches the teat, which Baby has sucked into a flat position, mother makes him get a new one. While waiting for the bottle, Baby arches his neck, looks in the direction of mother's face, and begins sucking noisily on his clenched fist.

When Mother moves him slightly, his hand falls out and he appears to be poised motionless in an interrupted movement. His body is tense. When he makes a few mouthing movements in the air, he seems more relaxed. He rolls his eyes in a backwards direction, arches his neck, scowls, and begins a muffled cry. He pushes his head back several times, while barely moving the rest of his body. When Baby resumes a light cry, mother rubs his tummy, but when the same intensity of crying continues, she gives him her breast, saying "probably there's nothing in there". We wait a few minutes until father returns with a new clean teat. Mother comments with relief that she can see how much baby drinks when he drinks from the bottle.

The couple joke about how indecisive they are about the baby's name. They say they have six weeks to name him. Father refers to the baby as "Algie" and recites a poem about the name given to the "bump on mother". Mother says he is number three in the family. It takes the couple two weeks to name the baby. This seems partially associated with their disappointment that, because his nose has been initially flattened from being pressed against the womb, he is not as attractive as the very perfectly formed parents hoped he would be.

Mother changes the baby, preparing him for sleep. She argues slightly with father, who wants Baby dressed differently for sleep. While changing the baby, mother says to the baby, "You're looking for the new visitor, aren't you. You can't get your eyes off her."

As I prepare to leave, mother tells me that she doesn't think she wants me to return. She is worried about my coming. She doesn't know why. I tell her that I appreciate how difficult it is to have so many new experiences with the baby and to have me present as well. Father says it will be all right for me to phone and come again the following week. Mother says she'd like more time to adjust to the baby first. She feels nervous about my being there. Father touches her arm and says, "By next week it will be okay, things will have settled more." I leave saying, "I'll phone. Thank you for the visit."

Observer in relation to the seminar

When I bring this first observation to the seminar, I am frightened of Mrs Bick. This fear superseded my original wish to understand the baby in his family. I, like Mother, have fears about the way in which I observe and describe my observations. I feel that Mrs Bick expects me to be a perfect observer, and there is too much nonverbal communication, like confetti, which must be caught, then knitted together into words and then paragraphs.

As I describe the initial visit, Mrs Bick asks questions which, on subsequent visits, act like a zoom lens of a camera to move the baby into very close, clear focus. Her questions are: "How is Mother holding the baby? Where is his head? How close to mother's body is he? Where is he looking? And what are his hands and legs doing when she changes position? What kind of movements or stillness do you see in the baby's body? Show us, we want to know." Through her questions Mrs Bick elicits more detailed descriptions of the quality of Mother's holding of Baby as well as additional comments on the various ways the baby "holds himself together". Each week the seminar begins with a reporter's summary of the discussion of the previous week, thus providing continuity between the observations. These are written in a literary style, telling the story of the family's emotional life evolving around the baby.

The observer in relation to the family

The seminar's interpretations of Baby's relationship to his parents have various effects on me. I feel that scales are being pulled off my defended "eyes", as Mrs Bick makes inferences about what I observe. I become eager to see in more detail how Baby and his parents are being held together. But at times I feel the seminar is exposing me too much. When Baby's experience has been fully described by Mrs Bick, I can hardly bear the experience of seeing him suffer. When Mother provides so little physical support for him, I tend to project into his experience my own infantile experience of not being emotionally held. I identify with Baby and become very critical of this mother, the bad mother of my internal world. I can barely restrain myself from saying, "He'll feel better if you hold him closer, if you hold his head."

When rashes develop on Baby's bottom, scalp, and face, I become ill and I have to miss a visit to the family. This illness occurs following a seminar in which Mrs Bick describes the baby's intolerable anxieties of spilling out and liquefying which are not being contained by Mother, leading to the baby's use of his skin as a kind of container. The interplay of my own infantile anxieties contained in earaches and colds as a child, stirred up by identifying with the baby's anxieties, results in my having a cold. This prevents me from seeing Baby.

Gradually, through the understanding and support of the seminar, I gain courage to work on the projections that I am carrying from the family members. This baby, in his damaged state, has been reluctantly accepted into his physically beautiful family. The mother is anxious about not being a perfect mother. I learn to "put myself in the shoes" of each family member, not just the baby's, and to remain sufficiently detached from my own anxieties to create a mental space to acknowledge my own anxieties and those projected into me by the parents. These include being experienced as the critic, the unwanted one, the competitive expert, the intruder.

A great deal of work on myself has to be done in order for me to be a good observer fully present with the baby and his family. When I do not do this work of keeping my feelings intensely alive and simultaneously thinking about them, I tend to cut off from intense emotional involvement. I become a wonderful video camera or I become a nanny, a second pair of helping hands to mother and baby. Then I can find emotional relief from the pain of being only an observer in the family without a child of my own, without the freedom to act in the capacity of a child psychotherapist, without the illusion of being a better mother than mother.

Finding new identities

Mother

Mother is obviously feeling very insecure. Not knowing what she should do to soothe the baby is unbearable. She worries, will her baby survive? Will she survive her baby? She responds to the advice of Father and the nurse by rebelling initially. Advice is felt as criticism of her not knowing what to do. She protects herself from feeling persecuted by the nurse by doing the opposite of the nurse's advice to wrap and hold the baby tightly. She shows her feelings of being persecuted by father by having him wash baby's teat the minute he touches it. Mother cannot invite her maternal grandmother, whom she admires, to her home until she, the mother, can show her that she is managing to care adequately for the baby. Mother's sense of persecution is transferred to her relationship with me and she tells me at the first visit, "Don't come back." When mother is bathing her 1-month-old baby and he cries, she feels that the cries mean she is not doing a good job mothering him. When she feels assailed by overwhelming demands to be a perfect mother, to have nothing for herself, these persecutory demands prevent her from using her good mothering capacities.

Clearly the baby's birth has precipitated in the mother a sudden and massive loss of identity. She is no longer the capable adult, the slim-figured woman, the competent librarian she was before the birth. She does not know who she is, having not yet acquired her identity as a mother. Her bewilderment and aching sense of loss of her old identity are joined to a realization of her total responsibility for this wee, helpless baby. Yet she feels utterly incompetent to the task. She feels herself to be like a newborn baby, suddenly vulnerable, exposed, unheld. By his responsiveness to Mother, his capacity to be comforted by her, Baby alleviates some of Mother's persecution. Mother introjects baby's responsiveness and appreciation towards her mothering. This helps her find an identity as a good mother. He does this by latching on to the breast, showing her that he wants and needs her and also by forgiving her quickly when she upsets him by not meeting his needs.

Father

In the initial weeks Father is more able than Mother to hold Baby closely and firmly in a way that enables Baby to feel secure. He is also able to be supportive to mother. At times, father's competence seems to be based on identification with good internal parents. At other times his competence seems to be based on projective identification with a "super-parent". This use of projective identification involves projecting his infantile anxieties into mother and baby and feeling an expert, an "old hand", at "mothering". On these occasions, being a good parent is out of competition with mother in order to cope with his infantile jealousy of baby frequently taking his place beside mother.

Father, like Mother, is also suffering a loss of identity and trying to find his place within the family. By the time baby is 3 weeks old, he has become more sensitive to his wife's insecurity about mothering and asks if she minds if he picks Baby up before he does so. However, as he allows her to be in the dominant position of being mother to baby, father's jealousy of Baby emerges. This is seen when Baby is being bathed at 3 months, with mother and observer in the bathroom. Father comes into the tiny bathroom carrying a photo of himself as a baby. He wonders if I think Baby looks like him. Now, feeling Baby is being cared for more than he is, feeling dropped and ignored, father defensively identifies with Baby. He says to me, "See my baby photo!"

Observer's identity

I say to the group, "I don't know how to make the baby 'more of a person' yet. Can you help me write in a manner that is more readable and vivid in its descriptive detail?" Mrs Bick says, "The mother is more central in your description. Baby is still sort of a strange object. His existence is not quite whole or secure in your descriptions. Can you infer some feeling when he cries, raises his arms, pushes his head back? What sort of facial expressions does he have?" I, like the parents, am having difficulty finding an identity for the baby and an identity as an observer. Mother has said, "The baby feels just like a lump, a stranger, an intrusion these first few weeks." That is just how I feel, initially, in the family home. I also feel inadequate for the seminar and for these anxious parents.

Seminar members' sense of identity

During this initial stage, the group—including me—remain virtually mute as though listening to a symphony orchestrated by Mrs Bick. No one would know that for all of us in the seminar this is our second baby observation. Many of the members have children, and most are qualified child psychotherapists. We have become passive recipients of Mrs Bick's wisdom about the early anxieties of mothers and babies. We are afraid to speak our thoughts, afraid to disagree with the thoughts of Mrs Bick. It is not only respect for Mrs Bick's understanding that causes passivity. It is also that we have settled for passive conformity with her thoughts, for we are afraid that if we are different, if we have separate identities, we might end up being "the unwanted baby". I do not think that this is an event peculiar to this seminar. Group passivity, in which members assume infantile dependence on being nourished by the expert, is perhaps one of the most daunting initial issues with which infant observation seminar leaders have to contend.

Concluding remarks on the first phase of the observation of baby until he is 4 months old

Mrs Bick discusses the baby, saying: "The baby is like an astronaut who has been shot into space without gravity, without a space-suit, with nothing to hold him together. This baby has a strong capacity for survival. This is related to his struggle *in utero*, when searching for a comfortable, secure, place in the womb. This is accentuated by mother, just before the birth, undergoing an emotional upheaval when her much loved grandfather dies. Baby is also an intelligent child and constitutionally strong. He is faced with a life-or-death struggle and, in the absence of a firm, containing mother, who can hold him both physically and psychically, he must rely on his own methods of coping with great insecurities."

In this early phase we see developing patterns in the baby's methods of protecting himself from anxiety. At 3 weeks, in an extremely frightening situation Baby, completely undressed, cries loudly, gets red in the face, kicks his legs rapidly, flails his arms stretched before him, passes wind, and defecates slightly. Non-stop movement is used by Baby, as if he is trying to hold himself together. He holds on to movement to prevent terror of a dead end. This does not succeed, and he seems to be "spilling out", with a flurry of uncontained emotions, sensual experiences, until Mother touches him. Then he becomes still, stops his crying, and momentarily has a calm facial expression. When Mother touches him, he is held, prevented from "falling to bits". Mother's touch derives its power from its significance as an adhesion, as a re-establishment of feeling that Mother is stuck on to him.

Beside non-stop movement, and stiffening of his back with his neck rigid and head thrust backwards, Baby holds himself from "spilling out" by curling up motionless. At 3 weeks, when his nappy is removed, his legs immediately curl to his chest. When Mother walks out of the room, it seems that his eyes, mouth, and diaphragm are all fixed still while he is holding himself tightly. When Mother returns, Baby opens his eyes and holds on to her face. While so held, his legs move in a gentle rhythm. This gentle movement of his legs when mother arrives suggests that Baby is able to let go of his own protective stillness, and link to mother in a way that allows him to move freely.

When Mother doesn't hold him firmly on her lap, Baby stiffens his body and back with his head pushing back. For example, at 4 months, Baby is lying untouched on Mother's lap. He pushes himself with his legs so that his back and neck are stiffly arched over mother's legs. His arms are also extended backwards. This wriggling backward is interrupted by short movements of restful attention on Mother's face. Stiffening of his musculature is baby's way of trying to make a stiff, holding, container for himself with all the energy he can mobilize. A colourful, striped, jump-suit, which always hangs nearby, is often used when Baby is not "emotionally held by mother". He stares at it intently, holding on to it with his eyes. Mrs Bick says that the organs—eye, mouth, ears, nose—serve as suction pads, like the mouth holding on to the nipple. At this early stage there is not much differentiation of the separate functions. They all seem to be suction pads for adhesion to hold oneself together.

There are two main methods by which Baby is able to hold himself together during these first four months. First, by using two middle fingers like a nipple to hold on to his mouth. This continued through his second year. For example, when Baby is 2½ months, Mother is changing Baby's nappies. As she removes his two fingers from his mouth to put on his jacket he begins to cry. He moves his arms agitatedly, kicking his legs, and moving his head about. Finally he finds his middle two right-hand fingers and sucks them while looking in my direction. Then he stops crying.

The other most satisfactory way of feeling held together is through listening to Mother's gentle, continuous, conversations with him. For example, at 4 months when Baby is being changed, he has his middle two fingers in his mouth when he lies on the changing mat. Mother begins talking to him. He releases his fingers from his mouth, breaks into a smile and then a laugh, with a kind of "goo-aah-hi" series of sounds when he becomes more excited as he waves his hand in flopping motions near his shoulder. As mother continues to talk to him he makes more sounds. He repeats some of her sounds. When Mother is talking to him, he does not need his fingers to feel securely held. The milk of Mother's love is going into him. He feels it and hears it. It is not he alone, but Mother and he are joined together like mouth with nipple inside. A genuine attachment, which requires time for Mother and Baby to get to know each other, has evolved.

When Mother is not too persecuted by Baby's cries, she is able to observe adequately what he wants and how he is. By the first month Baby has introjected some kind of internal holding mother and is able to relax his body and explore the world. For example, when he is 1 month, Baby's arm is wrapped close to his chest with his clenched fingers placed near his shoulder. His slightly bent legs stay still, with his toes slightly curled under. He sucks energetically. After about seven minutes at the breast, Baby extends his arm and gradually spreads his fingers like flower petals opening out. With his fingertips he gently moves along Mother's blouse and along her breast. Mother strokes his fingertips, squeezes them, and lets them go. He begins sliding his hand along Mother's breast in a very slow fashion. All this suggests taking in, in contrast to "hanging on" or "holding on to". This seems the beginning of Baby's exploration of his world, which is possible when he is emotionally held by mother.

In this first part of the chapter, I have given a detailed observation of Baby and his family in order to make a clear differentiation between his attaching himself to M other in a way that permits introjective experiences to take place (as in the example I just gave of the baby sucking on the nipple), and his "holding himself together" out of distress (holding his body very still, maintaining a stiff, arched back, holding on to the colourful jump-suit, holding on to his two right-hand fingers placed in his mouth).

An important aspect of these attempts by Baby to prevent catastrophe is that he is so frantically trying to hold himself together that no knowledge, no exploration of his world, no deepening relationship with his mother and father is possible. In this act of "holding on" in an adhesive way, no change is tolerated. Only repetitive sameness is accepted. If M other removes the fingers at this point, when Baby is using them to hold himself together, he is frantically distressed. In the course of Baby's development, as I described his putting his fingers in his mouth, I needed to begin differentiating his holding on to his fingers "for dear life" from his "sucking on" or "gently holding on" to the fingers with modified anxiety in a way that seems to be a re-creation of the experience of a good feeding breast.

We can admire babies who struggle to hold themselves together, but we also worry if they rely too much on their own attempts to care for themselves. A baby needs to feel secure enough to let go of his own protective methods, to face the uncertainty of a relationship with the mother. In the excerpt of Baby at 1 month at the breast, we see how, after about seven minutes of sucking at the breast, he seems to have sufficiently introjected Mother's attentive, emotionally holding, feeding to let go of his own bodily defences of stiffening of his hand and feet muscles. He then moves freely in his attempts to explore her.

When Baby can neither rely on mother's containment nor "hold himself together", his unpleasant experiences are expelled. This is through various orifices—spitting out from his mouth, defecating, projecting through his eyes, screaming or crying out, kicking out as if to kick out the unpleasant sensation, rapidly flailing his arms. This spilling out, or thrusting out, of unpleasant sensation needed to be differentiated from non-stop movement to hold the unintegrated self together. This differentiation was made by observing the expression on Baby's face together with the quality of the movements and the context in which he was behaving this way. For example, when M other stopped temporarily touching Baby while changing him, he may begin kicking. Depending on how anxious or angry baby was, he either began kicking wildly in fury or panic, or kicking forcefully to feel that his liquefying self was "held together" and alive, or he may have kicked in conjunction with the waving of his arms as a signal for Mother to pick him up. Hence, Mrs Bick would often say to me, "It's no good saying he is kicking—*how* is he kicking?"

Likewise, Mrs Bick would expect me in my observer capacity to begin to describe in detail and interpret the quality of Baby's crying, with a sensitivity similar to that of any mother who gets to know her baby well. I would need to describe the high-pitched cry of Baby in pain with a stomach-ache, the bellowing of a baby who is tired and gradually subsides into sleep, or the cry of the terrified infant who turns away from the mother when she tries to comfort him because his whole world has turned bad.

During times when noxious experiences are not expelled, Baby's body is used as a container, his bottom has a red rash, and his scalp has the flaky skin of cradle cap. This suggests that Baby's body can no longer tolerate the unpleasant tension he is experiencing. At this time the psyche becomes a sieve-like container, unable to retain distressing emotional experiences or to transform unpleasant sensations into emotional experiences that Baby can tolerate. Thus one sees how, in the first four months of life, the young infant is clearly filled with a great deal of anxiety that needs to be emotionally received and contained by the mother.

Getting established:
middle phase, 8–16 months

In this section, Baby's attempts to know about his world, and make sense of it, are highlighted.

Baby and his family: the book as breast

As early as 10 months, when   Baby is distressed Mother uses his interest in books to comfort him, instead of soothing him directly. For example, when Baby falls and begins crying, he is patted once by Mother, who then hastens to distract him: "Jeanne's here, she'll wonder why you're crying. Look, here's a book. Don't cry. It's nothing. There, there." In the instant that M   other hands him the book, Baby stops crying and carefully turns the pages. He talks incessantly, making sounds such as "de-de", which are similar to the sounds of the ducks he had in his bedroom mobile. He points at the pictures on the pages and says "derh" while looking up at me for a response. He smiles when he sees me looking at him. When he closes the book, he rubs the back and starts looking through it again. He pats some of the pages and crawls near the door to play peekaboo several times. He laughs as he shuts the door in our faces.

For Baby, his relationship with the book and all its wonders is symbolically linked with the relationship to the good internal breast, to his union with a loving mother and father reading to him. The book represents the treasure-house of all that a good loving mother provides—loving, talking, touching, thoughtfulness. He holds the book and pats it as though he possesses "the good breast". He is involved in it as he was involved in feeding intently at the breast. Then, in his peekaboo game, he works on his separation from his mother.

Knowledge used to allay anxieties about "broken connections"

Baby continues to resort to holding on to his two fingers in his mouth when extremely distressed, but as he grows older he relies more on his memory and intelligence as a means of holding himself together. He needs to know about what is happening, to know the routine of the family, to know about the spatial order of things in the house. Mrs Bick described how Baby holds on to the sameness of objects, the sameness of Mother's routine, the sameness of the observer in order to feel securely held. If objects change or are not in their proper place, if Mother's routine does not follow the sequence that he remembers and expects, then the world that Baby knows tends to collapse. His insecurity begins and increases, and then he greatly needs reassurance. Although he is a baby who acknowledges his dependence on a mother who provides a great deal of security, he has also learned to rely on himself, and his observation and attention are acute for everything.

When Baby is 9½ months, a few days after a clock has been removed from a box in a prominent position near the entrance to the sitting-room, he crawls near the box. He pauses below this empty box. Then he extends his right arm, later his left arm, pointing to the box while making sounds, "da [*pause*] da". He looks at me, then at the space where the clock was and repeats "da [*pause*] da". He then slowly crawls through the hallway. When M   other greets him and walks through the hall, he stops crawling and bursts into sharp cries. He is experiencing the inexplicable and worrying absence of the clock and trying to share his worry with his mother. Mrs Bick described the severe anxiety that arose in Baby because of this sudden change in the setting that included the familiar clock in its usual place.

However, according to Mrs Bick, Baby gradually has less need of adhesive identification as a protection against anxieties regarding unintegration or disintegration and changes. This security in Baby comes from having introjected Mother's containing presence, which creates an internal mental space. This internal space permits him to develop a gradually increasing capacity to elaborate on his emotional experiences through play. He is thus able to use talking, books, and games like hide-and-seek to re-create closeness to his parents and to work on his preoccupying anxieties about being dropped and lost, picked up and held. He is also able to use play to dramatize his phantasies of damaging and mending.

Mother became pregnant when baby was 10 months old. I shall give examples of themes in Baby's play activities which extend throughout most of Mother's pregnancy.

Play at 11 months :   Baby begins spilling milk and watching it fall on the floor. He throws pears on the floor and watches Mother retrieve them.

Play at 12 months: Baby finds a white spool-shaped man in the corridor, rolls it along the floor, catches it, bangs it on the floor, then begins talking to it. Later in his high chair, he smiles at me, drops the man, and looks at it on the floor. Mother retrieves it, and he bangs it against the high chair, throws it forcefully down, and then searches for it.

Play at 16 months :   A new edition to the former play routine occurs—baby throws a small horse on the floor, picks it up, kisses it, and throws it down again.

Activity at 16½ months :   Baby notices my bandaged finger. He touches it gently, then touches the hurt finger again very gently, saying "Ooh, ooh". Then he carefully bends down and kisses it. He tells his mother, "Jeanne, finger." His worries about the hurt finger are shown through his mentioning the hurt finger several times during my visit.

In these four observations during the time when Baby is 11 to 16 months old, a variety of emotional experiences are expressed by him. At 11 months it seems that Baby is experiencing   Mother's sense of being pregnant as something that makes him anxious. The spilling of the milk and the throwing of the pears, which requires mother to retrieve them, suggest that Baby is feeling unheld, dropped, and in response to these anxieties he is controlling mother to respond to him. He needs M other to reassure him that she will pick him up, hold him, and keep him in her mind. At 16 months, Baby himself retrieves the object he drops and kisses it in order to mend whatever is damaged.

Play is used by him not only to explore and master the conflicts in his external world, but also to work through his phantasies causing internal conflict. In his play we see that   Baby has a sufficiently internalized, good containing Mother which enables him to notice what is damaged externally. This external damage symbolizes what is damaged internally through his phantasized attacks. He then attempts to make reparation, partly through kissing of the male doll, but also through depressive concern for my damaged finger. Baby's noticing and feeling sorry about his destructive attacks, his wish to repair the damage, and his rebuilding of the internal breast or mother inside himself is part of the gradual process observed again and again in his play in subsequent observations.

The relationship of the observer to the family (middle phase, 8–16 months)

Mother feels abandoned by me on occasions when it is necessary for me to change the time of the visit. Through her behaviour, I become aware of how keeping to a regular time and length for our meeting provides containment for her. Breaking our routine of meetings disrupts our relationship. When I do change the times of our meeting, Mother, in her infantile transference to me, always responds by missing the next few meetings. She is simply not home when I arrive. Also, if I follow Baby out of the room in which Mother is also present, she feels neglected by me and responds by rejecting me. On the occasions when I phone to find out if Mother

will be available for the time agreed upon for later that day, she
indicates that she wants a "demand-feeding observer" by telling
me that the only time we can arrange to meet is just that moment,
right when I am phoning. In this way she communicates that she
does not want to be kept waiting.

Baby, meanwhile, is increasingly mobile and talkative. In his
mind, I am virtually part of his family. As early as 11 months, he
greets me with "Mummy, Daddy, Jeanne", and he frequently repeats these words during my visits.

Observer in relation to the seminar

I bring to the seminar my difficulties about Mother's apparent
rejection of me and Baby's engagement of me in his activities. I am
convinced that the observations continue only because of the seminar's understanding of what is going on between the family and
me. I am ready to stop the observations, because I keep feeling that
I am a nuisance and that that is why Mother isn't home when I
arrive. I can't acknowledge that Mother may be using me as a
container for her pain about being rejected. It is very difficult for
me to accept my importance to the family, particularly to Mother.
This is chiefly because I feel paralysed to do anything with Mother's dependence in her infantile transference to me. I can't interpret
the fact that she feels lonely and abandoned at home and deserted
by me. I can merely show her that I can withstand projections of
her feelings of being dropped. Mrs Bick also shows me the ways in
which I foster Mother's difficulties when I do not internally work
through any unvoiced criticisms of mother or I follow and watch
the baby too much rather than keeping a hovering attention on the
whole family at home. Later, Mother is able to tell me about her
loneliness, her sadness over her grandmother's death, and her difficulties and pleasure in being Baby's mother. These developments
in mother's relationship to me are possible only because the group
supports me and understands how I do have an important role for
mother even though I say very little.

I began the observations as a wooden statue, not engaging in
any activities with Baby. Later I discover that I have some joints

and can move. This occurs after Mrs Bick says, "Follow his lead. Don't initiate anything new. Hold what he gives you until he wants to take it away. Don't return it until he wants it back."

Baby comes up to me in many of my visits, to touch me and to say "bye-bye". Mother says, jokingly, that maybe he feels I only know how to say "bye-bye" to him. But in my silence I am still very present in his mind. Again, it is very difficult for me to understand how, just by being there, regularly, in an attentive way, without saying much, an observer can serve a useful function for a child. Gradually I become profoundly aware of how my silent understanding of mother is genuinely therapeutic. The seminar, by pointing out my usefulness as a psychic container for both Baby and Mother, then increases my guilt about planning to leave Baby soon after the new baby is born. The group's insistence on my usefulness intensifies a personal crisis in me: "If I am valuable to the family, and they have given me such a wonderful learning experience, how can I leave them? How can I, an observer, help a very young child understand that I am going to stop visiting him regularly?"

Traversing of catastrophic change: final phase, when baby is 22–32 months and the new baby is 1–10 months

"Every step in development requires a learning from experience and traversing of a catastrophic change."

Donald Meltzer (1986b, p. 12)

The seminar has now become smaller. At times I feel that I am demand-feeding the seminar. I am ready to stop the observations, but the group's interest in the new baby spurs me on. I decide to visit the family until they move away. "Eric"—the name I shall now give Baby—is 22 months. Mother tells me that she doesn't want me to visit any longer. The new baby is due in ten days' time. Being startled by mother's wish for me to stop, I have the nerve to ask her, "Can I come one more time, just to say goodbye? I'm not quite prepared for this to be the last visit." Mother reluctantly agrees.

Eric at 22 months :   When I arrive for the final visit, bringing a small glass bowl for Mother and Father,   Mother's eyes fill up with tears and she says, "Oh, but I don't want you to stop coming. I don't know what I was thinking when I told you to stop. Eric would miss you. You're somebody whom he knows comes to see him, and he's sad already with the new baby coming." When we agree to continue the observations, Mother says she is overwhelmed with so many things to do with the moving and everything, including the new baby. She kisses me and says she wants to go and put her glass bowl in a safe place where Eric can't reach it.

Eric meanwhile is saying, "Boat, where's my boat?" Mother says that she thinks he remembers that I gave him a present, too, a boat for Christmas.

This memory for his past experiences enables Eric to frequently join in the discussions that M other and I are having.

Eric at 22 months: In learning the word holiday, he interrupts, saying, "Beach, beach" and "Cuckoo, Cuckoo". Mother is astonished, saying, "Do you really remember that we were at the beach and there was a cuckoo in the house in which we were staying?" He smiles, delighted that mother understands, and he repeats with pleasure, "Cuckoo, cuckoo."

Mother is continuing to give meaning to his experiences. It is clearly important for Eric to be the centre of Mother's attention and mine. He is beginning to struggle over conflicts about the new baby. This is indicated by more frequent attacks on objects and relentless searches into the inside of objects. One could say that Eric would be doing this anyway at this age, but the change in his play suggests that he is clearly aware of the baby inside M other.

Eric at 22 months: In the kitchen, Eric is playing with a basket full of plums and tomatoes. He rubs them, holds them gently, squeezes them, and throws them, one by one, onto the floor. As he does this he says, "Tomatoes, plums, see Jeanne." After Mother picks them up and puts them back into the basket, he pats them once more and gently drops them on the floor again.

When Mother scolds him, he climbs up on to the stove, then on to a counter, and removes corks from the spice bottles. This is forbidden territory. He looks inside the bottles, replaces the corks, and looks alarmed when Mother removes him from the counter. He then runs to my handbag, lifts it up, and quickly puts it down and then asks me for a drink. Subsequently he reaches for a cup on the sink.

Later he climbs under the glass table where we are seated. While patting my leg and giggling, he calls up to us, "Hello Mummy, hello Jeanne." He then gets out from underneath the table and begins twirling around excitedly. Shortly he runs to get a puzzle which he brings to Mother saying, "Fix the puzzle, fix it Mummy."

Over the months Eric develops a capacity to bear feelings and hold experiences in his mind. He manipulates the objects in the house (the plums, the tomatoes, the corks, my handbag, the puzzle) in an exciting way, for he is endowing them with aspects of his internal world. He touches and drops the plums, then becomes concerned about the little one he has dropped out of the "basket Mummy". Out of curiosity about the contents of Mother's body, the new baby inside, he investigates the cork bottles and the space under the glass table. He is struggling with the wish to be the only one inside Mother's mind, beckoning for all her attention, asking her, "Can you let me inside?"

Then he beseeches Mother to help him put together the pieces of the puzzle with a bus and bus conductor inside. He hopes to fix the pieces together and wants Mother to help make his internal objects whole and good after his attacks, and he is reassuring himself that a good mother is there to help him. He is able to fix part of the puzzle himself and feel the pleasure of finding ways of putting the object back together, but then he can't complete the task. He demands, "Fix it Mummy."

Mrs Bick impressed us with her understanding of the toddler's severe crisis of identity when the new baby is born. "Eric is not simply experiencing jealousy," she said. "He doesn't know where he belongs." When he has a place in the social world outside the family it is slightly easier, but Eric is not yet in nursery. Initially, says Mrs Bick, he feels as aggrieved and misplaced as a partner does when a spouse has an affair. He is very worried: "How can I be M other's baby when this new baby sits there inside M   ummy and why am I not in there as well?"

My worry, of course, is: will the couple be able to fix things well enough for Eric so that he will not feel "in pieces" when   Mother and Father welcome home the new baby and place Eric in a new nursery? My concluding remarks show how Eric attempted to face the problem of changing from the position of being the only baby to being the "older brother". I include descriptions of how Eric's parents assisted Eric in his various stages of psychological adjust- ment to the new baby.

Being the baby

Eric at 25 months: The new baby, whom I shall call "Daniel", is 11 weeks old. While Mother is breast-feeding baby Daniel, Eric lies in the baby bouncer facing them while sucking his fingers. When Mother sternly tells him to get out, he forcefully throws the baby bouncer sideways at M other.

Later, when the new baby is put into Eric's former bedroom, Eric goes into his parents' bedroom, takes one of baby's blan- kets, and unsuccessfully wraps his teddy in it. When the blan- ket keeps falling off, as he picks up teddy he asks M   other to help, saying that he has to cover teddy or "he'll get pneumo- nia".

In Eric's mind there seems to be "a baby" who is clearly in danger of dying or falling ill. His thought about an ill baby is linked with his anxieties about wanting to take the new baby's place. It is also connected to Eric's sense of being left "out in the cold" while the new baby is being fed.

Splitting loving and hating feelings

At times Eric cannot manage the intensity of the conflict be- tween his loving and his hating feelings. He then resorts to split- ting the hostile feelings off into various relationships, in order that somewhere he can preserve a good loving relationship.

Eric at 26 months: Eric begins nursery school. He returns home to enjoy bathing under M other's care. He says, "I love you Mummy." On this same occasion he will not come near me as he usually does, and he refuses Mother's request to "say good-bye to Jeanne". This is unusual.

Eric at 28 months :   Eric is very nice to baby, but he is increasingly defiant to Mother, saying "No" to each of her requests for him to have a bath and to leave his toys in the play area.

Eric at 28 months: Eric gets cross with Mother for giving baby a toy she won't let Eric have. When M other attempts to wash him in the bath, Eric refuses to let her. He says, "Jeanne, wash me." When I reply that I shall watch him, he washes his body excitedly, while naming all the parts of his body.

Jealousy of the new baby spoiling all his relationships

There is a change in his behaviour now, for Eric no longer restrains the expression of his hostility to the baby by directing all hostility to Mother or the observer. However, his physical attacks on the baby are very tentative and clearly marked with some respect for the fact that baby should not really be hurt.

Eric at 28 months :   When Mother arranges a bath for Eric and his young brother, Eric throws his stuffed rabbit at Daniel, and then he sips some bath water and spits it at Daniel's face. Eric then quickly covers baby Daniel's face with a wet facecloth. Later Eric is obviously concerned about doing damage when he picks up a tiny plastic frog and tellsMother, "The eye is out." In an attempt to make things better, Eric gives baby a little plastic toy saying, "Daniel likes to eat it."

Watching baby suck on the toy provokes Eric's jealousy of baby at the breast. When M other attempts to give baby a plastic barrel, Eric cries out, "I want it, Mummy." He shouts until Mother takes the toy away from baby and gives it to Eric. But it is not the toy that Eric wants, for when M   other gives baby another toy, Eric cries and screams, with a desperate, piercing sound, "I want it Mummy."

The toys symbolize all Mother's emotional riches, which are now also bestowed on the new baby. Eric is riddled with jealousy of baby receiving a share of Mother's love. When Mother takes Eric out of the bath, he refuses to stand. Instead, he raises his legs, causing him to drop in a heap on the carpet. Then he begins biting the carpet and making all sorts of "gooh-gooh" sounds. After Mother dries him, Eric hurriedly runs for the comfort of his father's lap, which is free of the new baby.

> *Eric at 28 months*:   Eric rests his head against his father's shoulder while sucking forcefully on his middle two fingers. Father begins reading a bedtime story that Eric usually enjoys. Eric cannot focus on the pictures, for he keeps looking across the room at mother feeding baby.

Eric's relationship to the good internal mother usually allows him to maintain an avid interest in storybooks. However, here we see that having Father's attention does not succeed in blotting out Eric's jealousy or sufficiently mitigating his sense of loss when he sees the new baby feeding at Mother's breast. Eric's experience of a loss of identity as Mother's baby as well as his jealousy of the new baby at the breast interferes with his pleasure of looking at his books and being with Father.

Projective identification with a grown-up daddy

Father is delighted to have a more clearly defined role—to take care of Eric while Mother cares for the new baby. However, Father tends to push Eric to use his intelligence to do things that are far beyond his current knowledge or capacities. Eric also has a strong wish to be big, like Daddy. This wish is entertained, in part, to avoid his infantile jealousy of the baby.

> *Eric at 29 months* :   Father announces to me that he and Eric have put together every single one of the many puzzles that Eric has. Eric has fixed up every single one of the pieces of a two-foot-long Noah's Ark puzzle by himself. Now, as he does it again, he says proudly to us, "I'm doing very well." He is delighted about being an older child who has skills, who can do

things that baby can't do. "It is not simply jealousy which prompts his activity. Being capable like Daddy means he has an identity separate from that of baby's identity", says Mrs Bick.

Father sings the alphabet song with Eric and shows him some letters of the alphabet. Eric correctly picks out the letter for baby's first initial. But then Father spends fifteen minutes trying to help Eric learn how to tell the time on a puzzle clock. When Eric can't tell the time, Father gets impatient with him, saying "Oh, I give up." Eric is totally crestfallen. He feels lost. He becomes quiet and sheepishly says, "I can't remember." He rubs his head very worriedly. Then he throws all the puzzle pieces composing the clock in a disorderly pile.

Repeatedly Mrs Bick emphasized the acuteness of Eric's anxieties regarding losing his identity as a clever, important person in his parents' eyes in order to differentiate himself from the new baby. If Eric can't be the boy who does very well, knowing things like Father, he feels he is nothing, he fails, he becomes like a baby again. He becomes miserable with the fear that there is no place for his "baby self" because a new baby has taken his place. However, a while later, Eric tries to get out of his vulnerable position of being a baby who doesn't know how to do things. He recruits me as an ally to observe his "big boy like D addy" activities. This time his activities are musical and physical rather than intellectual.

> *Eric at 29 months* :   When Eric hears M other talk about her friend who sings, Eric struts around singing, "la, la, la". He then says, "I'm kicking my ball. It's a big ball." Hearing Mother offering coffee, he demands, "Mummy, I want a cup of coffee." When mother says, "You don't like coffee, do you? Have some Ribena or juice", he answers, "No." Then he firmly repeats his request, "I want coffee."

Here we see Eric's attempts to possess and control Father's grown-up capacities to tell the time and fix a complicated clock puzzle. He ignores his own preferences, saying that he wants what Father drinks—coffee. At the same time Eric disowns and projects his baby feelings into baby on mother's lap. Only baby is to have the baby position of wanting M other's milk, or Ribena or juice. Eric

projectively identifies with Father in order to postpone a sense of
loss of identity and confrontation with jealousy that his baby self
experiences in relation to the new baby.

Being "baby" with mother

When Eric has some time alone to talk and play with Mother, he
introjects this satisfying experience and is then able to share her
with the new baby.

> *Eric at 29 months:*   Eric has spent some time in the kitchen with
> Mother before she leaves and returns. When she stoops down to
> wipe up some coffee spilled on the floor, Eric seeing her at this
> level quickly asks to sit on her free leg. Mother allows Eric to do
> this. Squatting before me with a child on each knee she laughs
> and says, "Aren't we a spectacle?"

My immediate response is to think how dramatically Mother has
changed since we first met. She wasn't able to respond to Eric's
requests to be picked up when he was 1½ years, but now, although
Eric barely realizes it, she is a mother who does have space for two
babies on her lap. It is clear that Eric is grateful to Mother for being
a good mother to him. His relationships with Father and with me
have assisted him in surviving the pain of accepting the arrival of
his baby brother, Daniel.

Allowing coupling to take place

> *Eric at 29 months:*   Later, when I'm watching Eric in the garden,
> he notices a small yellow flower that has dropped off a bush. He
> brings it to me saying, "That's for you." Then he looks on the
> grass, saying, "I'll get a flower for Mummy." When we go
> inside the house, I give both flowers to   Mother, but Eric says,
> "No, that's for Mummy. That's for Jeanne." He wants to kiss me
> goodbye.

In the past, Eric's wish to kiss me goodbye has occurred mainly
when baby is in   Mother's lap and Eric is turning away from
Mother, wanting to distance himself from Mother with baby. This

visit is different in that he is able to keep affectionate and distinct relationships with both Mother and me. He is very sensitive to the beauty of the breast and to his greedy wishes to possess it completely and control it. Here though, he wants me and his mummy each to have a flower. He seems identified with the internal mother who has space for both baby Daniel and himself. He has begun to see the possibility of having something for himself without damaging the new baby, or Father, or M other's relationship with me. As mouth and nipple, Mother and baby, and Mother and Father, begin to remain linked together in his mind, Eric wants me to put the flower back on the plant. He wants me to help him to bring things together and keep them connected.

Symbolic play used to enlist parent's help with anxiety-laden feelings

When the family move to a new city, Eric is quite unhappy, particularly without his playgroup friends. The strain of being without a diversion from his baby brother Daniel, and Daniel's relationship with the parents, is obvious.

Eric at 32 months and Daniel at 10 months   :   Baby is crawling behind Eric wherever he goes and trying to touch everything that Eric is playing with. Eric says, "Go away, it's mine!"

Then Eric becomes anxious about his hostility towards baby. When baby goes near the staircase, Eric tells father, "Watch because baby will fall down the stairs." Father laughs and sits on the staircase while Mother prepares the children's bath. Eric then goes to his bedroom and looks out of the window. He exclaims, "Why, there is a dinosaur out there. Come look." Father replies, "Oh no, I can't, because I'm watching to make sure the baby doesn't fall down the stairs." Eric then gets teddy from his bed, leans near Father, and throws teddy down the stairs. Father says, "Oh, poor teddy". Eric laughs excitedly. He orders Father to "go and get it". Father says, "No, I'm watching the stairs to see baby doesn't fall." Eric says, "I'll go and get it." He climbs over Father and asks, "See? I'm not going to fall, am I?" He retrieves teddy and takes him to the bathroom, where he hides him under the bathtub. Returning to   Father and me, he tells us, "There's a dinosaur out there. It's very big. It's sitting in the middle of the road. It has two teeth. See how big it is." He points to the road outside. Then Eric tells me he is going to hide. While hiding under the parent's bedcovers he calls out, "I'm hiding from the dinosaur, Daddy." When Father comes into the room he wants Father to hide too.

In these activities Eric is striving to get Father to notice how, when he is left without Mother, he feels he is falling. Eric tries to distract father from protecting baby, and he tempts Father to concentrate on him. When Father doesn't take seriously enough Eric's wish to be protected, Eric is subjected to the frightening dinosaur. The dinosaur embodies combined bad internal parents—Mother joined with Daddy in a union filled with his projections of hatred towards the new baby and the couple giving birth to him. Eric's own sadistic wishes against the parental couple turn them into a monstrous dinosaur, revengefully coming back to attack him. In his staircase play, the teddy is used to personify Eric's vulnerable self and his fears of being the annihilated baby. A secret protected life for his "fragile self" is sought through his hiding of teddy, symbolizing his baby self.

On the same day, following this elaborate play activity, Eric is able to relate to his hostilities and fears with more depressive concern than persecution:

Eric at 32 months :   Having struggled to take away baby's toys in their joint bath, Eric returns to Father to show him a slight cut on his hand. He then finds an army tractor, rolls it in front of me, and says, "The wheels are broken, fix it, Jeanne." I put the wheel on, but when the tractor doesn't roll, he takes it to Father. Then he calls loudly to me from the other room, "Daddy is fixing it. I'm helping." He sounds very pleased.

One of the striking features here is how Eric tries to enlist his good external parents and me to help him with his fears. These fears are related to his need to be held more securely, particularly in the face of his jealous attacks to his damaged self, the damaged internal brother, and the parents.

But it is not simply jealousy with which Eric is struggling. Mrs Bick felt that we must penetrate underneath the concept of jealousy to understand how deeply Eric feels that the new baby takes away a sense of his own identity. When he is the only child with his parents, Eric has a sense of his own identity. Alone with his parents, Eric has a sense of being their child whom they love. When he is coupled with baby, joined with baby in play, in the mutual bath, or looking at baby feeding on Mother's lap, Eric loses his sense of identity as "the baby". He is not yet certain about his new identity, that of an older child, the big brother who doesn't need to be just the same as baby, or just the same as Father, to have what the parents provide for him.

The ending of the seminars

Throughout her discussion of the couple's transition to the parenthood of not one, but two, children and Eric's move from being the only child to sharing the family with a new baby, Mrs Bick had stressed the development of a sense of identity, and the loss of a sense of identity which creates profound anxieties. When she discussed how Eric was not yet certain about his new identity, I realized that I and other members of the seminar were also making a transition. Near the end of the observations, Mrs Bick had entered a nursing home and was ending her career when she completed the seminars. Despite her physical frailty and sense of impending death, with the utmost sensitive attention and love she had nourished our development through her illumination of the inner world of the baby.

I was painfully aware that now our sense of identity of being "her students" was also changing. Each of us was developing within ourselves to find our own sense of identity as teachers of infant observation. We would not necessarily have to be "the same" as Mrs Bick to feel that we were using our own insights in fostering the development of infant observation. When members of the group meet today, twenty years later, they still speak of "Mrs Bick's seminar" and what an important growing experience we had through being present with Mrs Bick. In touch with her own anxieties of dying, she described with such sensitivity and comprehension the baby's and the mother's early infantile anxieties, as we followed the minute details of the process of verbal and nonverbal interaction between the infant and his family.

Conclusion

The family's move marked the end of the observations, and the end of the seminar with Mrs Bick. The ending of my visits to the family, particularly after such a lengthy observation period, provoked many questions regarding how to end the observations. I wondered, "How do I leave the family? I don't feel that it is appropriate to switch immediately from the role of observer to friend of the family." This is an inclination that frequently arises at the end of observations. I decided to visit the family occasionally, with several months elapsing before I visited as a possible friend, rather than as an observer. I imagined that, after some months had passed, there would be time for my role as an observer—with all the infantile transferences it carries from the mother—to be stored as a memory, leaving space for what, if anything else, could then later emerge between me and the family.

My aim in writing this chapter was not to trace the complexities of the baby's emotional development into childhood. Instead, I hope to have highlighted some of the central preoccupations with early infantile anxieties, in particular the fear of disintegration and loss of identity, which are central to Mrs Bick's contribution to the study of infants. Through her devotion to observing and understanding the child and the parents, Mrs Bick fostered our own wishes to participate in a concerned way in the seminar. I frequently reminisce about Mrs Bick. I would like to dedicate this chapter to her, for her help in bringing to life in me, in a vivid and meaningful way, the full impact of the experiences of a baby new to the world and of the parents new to the task of rearing him.

Acknowledgements
I am grateful to Dr Shirley Waugh of Australia and others who took many detailed notes for the seminars with Mrs Bick.

CHAPTER SIX

Mrs Bick and infant observation

Joan Symington

M rs Bick loved babies, children, and psychoanalysis.
During the war she worked in a nursery in Manchester.
She noted the agitation and disturbed behaviour of the
children. She found that if she gave them empty tins and a few
pebbles to play with, the children spent the time putting the pebbles into and out of the tins and their behaviour settled down. In
other words, she was always well aware of problems of containment and its lack. This derived also from remembered early childhood experiences of the sudden loss of the feeling of security. [1] On
thinking about these experiences later in life, she came to realize
that feeling held together may be a very precarious and relative
matter, which could easily be upset by a sudden shock.

I first met her when I began my analytic training at the British
Psychoanalytical Society. She was to take our infant observation
seminars, and this was a preliminary discussion with her about

---

This chapter is based on "The Suction Tentacle", in S. Alhanti & K. Kos-
toulas (Eds.), *Primitive Mental States: Across the Lifespan, Vol. 1.*   Hillsdale, NJ:
Jason Aronson, 1997.

[1] Esther Bick, personal communication in 1979.

this. When we got to the question of how to find a suitable baby, she wondered if my general practitioner might help. At that stage I had no GP as I had not yet registered with one, and I told her so. She contradicted me saying, "But of course you have a general practitioner." I was a bit nonplussed by her certainty, and mentally I made a note that she was a typical know-all Eastern European matriarch. I was not the only one to experience this character trait of hers.

Nevertheless, when the infant observation seminars began I quickly came to realize that I was in the presence of someone with a phenomenal mind, who was able to observe afresh and think independently and, through this and her love of children, had come to a profound understanding of the infant mind not only in babies but in children and adults. Thus her know-all quality could be seen as a carapace—to use her own terminology—but in many ways a gossamer-thin carapace that by no means detracted from her exceptional ability.

In these seminars she began by showing us in great and convincing detail from the material brought by one or other of us students how the new mother feels totally responsible for her baby, so much so that she has a feeling of imprisonment. The new mother has also lost her identity. She no longer feels competent. She used to be someone, in her job, in her marriage, in her social life. She feels, therefore, very uncertain and, in this sense, is in exactly the same position as her baby, who has not yet found his sense of identity. The mother feels incompetent in her new task and in many other areas of her life. She no longer knows who she is. In some ways she feels like a little girl confronted with a real baby instead of just a doll. In that she is suffering a considerable loss, she is depressed. Her depression manifests itself in her partial withdrawal from her baby. She gives the baby her breast to feed from but withholds herself. She may hold the baby in her arms and lap but not hold him with her mind. This is the mother's part-object relationship with her baby. Mrs Bick demonstrated this again and again in each infant observation. In other words, depression in the new mother seems to be universal.

She showed how the observer identified with one or the other— that is, with either the depressed mother or with the infant who is missing out on his mother's full attention. Some students would feel indignant on the baby's behalf and angry with the mother, perhaps an echo of their own resentment at deprivation. Others would feel sorry for the mother in her enormous task for which she felt so ill-prepared. Some would want to give her concrete reassurance or support, others would want to step in on the baby's behalf. In all cases it was necessary to reflect on these matters, to recognize what one was experiencing, so that in coming to an understanding no action was then necessary.

The sense of being totally responsible for the baby is likely to make the mother feel persecuted. Is she doing the right thing? Is she good enough for the baby? Will it survive her care? She watches to see how the baby responds. If the baby sucks well, she is reassured that she is a good mother. This is why mothers are preoccupied with the baby's weight. If the baby is gaining weight, this is concrete proof that her mothering is adequate. She feels very uncertain of her breast milk. What she sees of it looks very thin in comparison with cows' milk. She isn't able to see how much the baby is getting, unlike with a bottle-feed.

If the baby goes on crying and can't be comforted, the mother feels full of persecutory guilt. To get away from this feeling she looks for concrete reasons for the baby's distress—wet or dirty nappy, hunger, tiredness, wind, colic. To attribute the baby's distress to one of these gives the mother much-needed relief.

Similarly if the baby becomes ill or develops a rash, the mother feels that it has occurred through her failure. She will be very sensitive about anything that could be taken as criticism of her—that is, her own skin is raw. She may ask the observer to leave so as not to have a witness to what she experiences as her failure. If the husband picks the baby up and it stops crying, while this at some level may be a relief to all, the mother may feel more persecuted that he can comfort the baby but she cannot.

If the baby is easygoing and tolerant, it is much easier for the mother. She is reassured and grows in confidence every time the baby is relieved or pleased. When the baby smiles and can show pleasure in other ways, this is of great mutual benefit.

Through the experience of ongoing weekly observation, the observer is able to see how the relationship between the baby and the mother gradually develops and strengthens. In this interaction, when she can feel that the baby needs her, the mother finds her

new identity as mother and, in this new identity, feels held together, contained.

To focus now more on the baby, Mrs Bick showed how a young
baby often feels himself to be in an unintegrated state. In this state
the baby looks like jelly, trembles or moves in a disorganized way,
or has attacks of hiccups or sneezing. She showed the baby desperately sticking to the nipple, unable to let go, and perhaps even
unable to suck. Before there is any concept of three-dimensionality
or of an inner space, anxiety is dealt with by finding an object to
stick to, by adhering to a surface with the force of a suction disc.
Once there is a concept of an inner space, anxiety propels an attempt to get right inside this space in order to feel held and safe.
The sticking stage occurs before there is an idea of an internal space
and so it occurs also before Klein's stage of splitting and projective
identification. The latter, at this early stage, is just a forward movement, an attempt to contact a surface. Melanie Klein (1932), following Freud, said originally that first the death instinct is deflected
outward very early in life so that it becomes an external threat and
therefore more manageable. It is projected out into something, into
the world. Mrs Bick is talking of a stage before this, before there is
any idea of an object with a space inside it.

The anxiety at this stage is a terrifying one of the self not being
held together but in constant danger of spilling out into endless
space where one would be lost forever. The skin is felt to be the
only thing that holds the parts of the self together, and it is felt to be
a very fragile and precarious holder, liable at any moment to be
perforated or torn. She painted various images of the self as a jelly,
shivering with terror in its unheld state. Safety is adhesion to a
surface. There must be no movement, as this would mean that the
adhesion was not safe.

It is not only in a tactile way that sticking can occur. It can also
be done with other sensory modalities—sticking with the eyes,
ears, or nose for example. The baby might be seen with his eyes
glued to the door through which his mother has just vanished, or,
with his ears, he may be sticking to the sound of her voice in the
next room. The importance of the sticking for safety is that nothing
else can happen at the same time. It is an all-or-nothing activity. In
this sense, it is one-dimensional—if the object disappears, life ends.
The object to which the baby sticks holds the attention, and it is this

holding of the attention that provides the temporary feeling of containment. This object is briefly experienced as a skin.

Mrs Bick likened this primitive projective process to an amoeba protruding a pseudopodium, on the end of which there is a suction disc that then sticks to the nearest surface. Or the eyes or ears are felt to be suction pads that can stick. The mouth holding on to the nipple could be sticking to it. At this primitive stage there is not much differentiation between all these ways of adhering to the object. While sticking assuages the fear of uncontrollable spilling out, it effectively stops any interaction with the object. It provides absolute continuity by contiguity. This absolute continuity is important in giving a sense of a continuous skin that has no hole or rents through which spillage could occur.

A similar sense of continuity is provided by the baby engaging in continuous movement—for example, by kicking with the legs when he is anxious. The idea is that if the movement does not stop, then no gaps can occur. Mrs Bick also called this the "J-model", after a patient who spent much time in her sessions engaged in drawing round and round a double-sided letter J (Bick, 1986). The same patient used to write across a sheet of paper until she came to the edge, when the writing would suddenly turn down vertically as though it had slipped over the edge of a cliff. Always, this is the anxiety—that of coming to an edge or a gap or hole through which spillage could occur. It is very common for people to have a sudden sense of falling just before sleep comes. This is a fleeting contact with the primitive anxiety. In adults as well as children, this continuous movement can often be seen—for example, when someone paces up and down or continually fiddles with some object or talks non-stop.

What may seem like the opposite of continuous movement is a third way of coping with catastrophic anxiety, and this is a holding still through tensing the muscles. If everything is frozen, nothing can spill or tear. A baby may suddenly freeze, as though in terror.

As this terrifying primitive anxiety is universal, babies all have these defences, but the amount to which they are resorted to depends on the ability of the mother to help the baby during its states of anxiety. If she is able to do this, if she can enable the baby to feel held together, these defences against anxiety become less prominent. The mother may not be able to hold the baby together adequately. This may derive from herself or arise from the infant's attacks on her. He may have torn her containing psychic skin.

Feeling held together means feeling that the self or parts of the self are safely held by a psychic skin. Defects in this skin may be revealed as actual skin problems. Mrs Bick said that the prototype of this containment is the nipple inside the mouth. I think that by this she meant that this is the most centring thing for the baby, the centre of its new world, so to speak, the mouth being the gateway to its mind and the nipple being the link to the outside world. Nipple-in-mouth is the prototype on which countless other holding situations are based. Thus, for example, the hand is an extension of the holding mouth. The baby can feel held together by holding something in his hand, perhaps his other hand or his foot. Basic inner security depends on the establishment in the mind of this prototype nipple-in-mouth holding.

When there is insufficient holding by the caregiver, the baby resorts to these defences more and more. They then become in-grained and form a pseudo-protective layer, or second skin, as Mrs Bick calls it. This tough outer layer hides an extremely fragile skin underneath. In this way, it is like a tortoise shell or carapace. The toughness is often encouraged by the parents—for example, a boy baby may be encouraged to be tough, to throw himself around, to not feel pain, to engage in continuous movement, because this reassures the parents that he is not only surviving but that he is lively. Children diagnosed with attention-deficit disorder are often like this. They cannot stop. They have had insufficient holding by the caregiver, for whatever reason. They may have been very diffi-cult to hold because of extreme intolerance to anxiety, or their parents may not have had the necessary experience inside them to enable them sufficiently to contain their baby's anxiety. So they are literally suffering from a deficit of attention.

This second skin may be constructed of a continuous activity such as talking. There are people who cannot stop chattering, be-cause they hold themselves together in this way. Others are forever busy; to stop means disaster. These activities have become in-grained and automatic and are part of the character structure.

The cardinal fact about the second-skin activities is that with them the baby can hold himself together. He no longer has to rely on anyone else. He feels he cannot risk doing this. He has to do it himself. This means that a baby may show great intelligence and skill in certain psychomotor tasks and mental abilities. Bick described an infant of 10 months who was so adept at doing things for himself that when he wanted music he could put the needle onto the gramophone record in an exact mimicry of his mother. These modes of survival, even though restrictive of human relationships, do promote development of certain abilities.

There is, of course, between the mother and baby adhesion in the form of stroking, which contributes both to body image and to the feeling of integrity. This is not defensive adhesiveness. Similarly when the baby reaches out and is met by the mother, who grasps or touches his outstretched limb, talks to him, and makes eye contact, this all has an integrating effect. Maria Rhode (1997b) has said that meaning must develop in the first instance in the mother's mind, with the coming-together of physical and mental experience. If, however, the baby's reaching out is not met by a response on the part of the mother, then sticking occurs instead.

The sticking also plays a non-defensive role in joining the parts of the self together, which I shall elaborate later in one of the following examples.

A 9-week-old baby, having just been dried after her bath, began to cry when she was put onto her back but stopped when she saw her mother's breasts uncovered as the mother washed her nipples. She stared at the breast. The baby was using her eyes to stick to the breasts. When the breasts were covered again, she trembled and then cried. When the baby was put down on her back, she felt exposed and unheld. The exposed ventral surface of the body feels vulnerable in comparison to the back and triggers an agoraphobic anxiety. She cried to try to expel this anxiety but when she saw the breasts and stuck to them with her eyes, she immediately felt held and stopped crying. Incidentally, Bick said that using the breasts to stick to in this way is unusual. The trembling that occurred when the breasts were covered indicated that she felt dropped and unheld. She then actively did something to help herself: she cried.

A second baby was seen during feeding to be staring at the mother's face with great intensity while stroking her hand and sucking strongly. In this case, a part of the baby—her eyes—

were desperately clinging, while other parts could take in and relate. A third baby, at 7 months, was lying on her back, moving her arms up and down. She smiled when she saw the observer, but while doing so she dropped the toy she had been holding. She froze, her movements stopped, and she stared in front of her absolutely immobile, her eyes in a fixed unblinking stare. Sticking with the eyes in order to cling to an object is quite different from taking an object in with the eyes.

Sticking goes together with learning by mimicry. The subject becomes the same as the surface to which it sticks. Thus, when a baby adheres with its back to a hard surface, it creates a rigid back. The child who is sticking onto the mother makes the same movement as the mother. This mimicry learning occurs before there is any mental space, so it occurs without thought. It is resorted to in times of stress.

I now want to give a rather long example to illustrate sticking being used in a non-defensive way or in the service of development. This example also illustrates Mrs Bick's remarkable capacity to grasp the relevant points and use them to bring alive the personality of the child described. It has been said that her ability to do this had a poetic quality displayed only by those who love life intensely.

> From very early on, it could be seen that this baby held on for a long time before suddenly bursting out with distress. The mother was gentle with the baby, and Mrs Bick thought that one facet of her gentleness was fear of the baby's violence, so that she was unable to hold her firmly enough. The baby also held back because she too was afraid of damaging the mother with her violence. So the two of them could not come together in a firm, penetrating, holding way—that is, nipple in mouth— in case the mother was destroyed. The only way the mother and baby could be put together was by sticking and mimicry. There was no basis of nipple-in-mouth holding. In her early weeks of life, the baby was seen to hold the teat of the bottle in her mouth for a long time without sucking. In other words, her need for holding was far greater than her need for food, and she tried to meet this need by sticking to the teat. Weeks later she was still

not able to get her fingers into her mouth because she had not yet established a sufficiently stable mental image of the nipple-in-mouth holding. She therefore developed a very rigid carapace.

During one observation when the baby was asleep, she remained absolutely immobile except for one brisk movement of her left leg, which she lifted up suddenly and then let fall again. This movement was striking in that it seemed to be confined to only one limb, as though the leg were independent of the rest of the body. Mrs Bick said that the baby was protecting herself against waking up, that every part of the body was separate, not joined together, so the waking up was confined to one leg while the other parts stayed asleep. When there is no mimicry, no sticking is possible; therefore, there is no sticking together of body parts.

She pointed out that the mother also very quickly lost her own sticking together. This could be seen when she washed the baby. It was a disjointed baby that she washed. She meticulously washed an eye, an ear, an arm, a leg in a disjointed fashion, and so absorbed was she in this activity that she did not speak for twenty minutes. During this time the baby was on her lap in a precarious position, but the mother was oblivious to this. This absorption in the task was the mother's carapace. She was not aware of a whole baby. Her fear that the baby would die was so great that she saw the baby as separate parts. The same behaviour can be seen in doctors who defend themselves against the fear of death by treating parts of the patient, not the whole person. The baby's carapace was manifest when the mother lifted up one of the baby's legs. The whole body lifted as well, because the baby was holding herself so stiffly. So you see that although the baby's body parts were not joined up mentally speaking, the thick second skin or carapace she had constructed for the purpose of holding herself together covered up this fact by a thick layer of stiffness. So we have a baby with a carapace to hold herself together in the absence of internal nipple-in-mouth holding and a mother, too, who has a carapace manifested in her ability to be totally absorbed and cut off to her baby's distress.

The following sequence describing the baby waking illustrates sticking being used in a non-defensive way. From being asleep, the baby sighed, moved her legs, and then lifted both arms up, slowly opening the fingers of both hands, bending each finger one after another and then straightening it out. Next she brought her hands to her face and touched her cheeks, ears, and eyes. Finally her head and neck stretched and then her legs. She made a noise like "ha", with her eyes still tightly closed. When her father spoke to her, she put both hands on her face and rubbed her eyes, which then gradually opened.

Mrs Bick said that by touching the various parts of her body, she was sticking to each part and was then able to come to-gether, come to life, and wake up. This touching is the bringing together, the mimicry learning, under the aegis of the life in-stinct. The repeated sticking contact, including rubbing the eyes, stuck the parts of her body together.

The baby who touches successive parts of her body in waking herself up is putting the bits together by successive touching, like a gentle tactile roll-call of the different parts. This is also a mimicry of the mother's armoured way of washing her, one part after another, as though the baby were in bits.

Under the life instinct, each reaching out and sticking of the baby is an alive contact that allows separation as opposed to the narcissistic immovable sticking where all is fused. Mrs Bick made this distinction, implying that even though the child is not being emotionally held together, there is life enough to go on trying to put the bits together.

There is a difference between, on the one hand desperately holding the parts of the self together through sticking and, on the other, a recognition and acceptance of the scattering, the "in-bits" state of mind, together with a wish to keep in communication with the dispersed parts by successively touching them. The ability to do this indicates that there is beginning to develop the concept of a container in which the self and its scattered parts are held.

A borderline psychotic young man, after some years of analysis, had begun a course on film and television production tech-niques. In one of the classes he saw himself on camera and was dismayed to see how little, scattered, and "un-cool" he looked. His teacher told him not to try to control the situation but to let it all happen. He did so, and by acknowledging his state of fragmentation he felt held.

Mrs Bick had a remarkable capacity for presenting her ideas in such a way that, each time, they appeared vibrant and new. She always left a door open for future developments. Sometimes she seemed to be presenting a point of view contrary to something she had said previously, but what finally emerged from this apparent contradiction was an enlarged understanding. There is something in this that reminds me of the touching of successive points to bring something to life, like touching different parts of the multifaceted whole bringing enriched understanding.

The baby holding himself together is very different from the baby using the mother in a way that allows introjection to take place. Jeanne Magagna gave an example in chapter 5 of a baby relating to the mother in an introjective way—that is, not having to rely on himself. "After about seven minutes at the breast, Baby extends his arm and gradually spreads his fingers like flower petals opening out. With his fingertips he gently moves along M oth-er's blouse and along her breast. Mother strokes his fingertips, squeezes them, and lets them go. He begins sliding his hand along Mother's breast in a very slow fashion." All this suggests taking in from the mother rather than a holding himself together. He felt held by her and was able to take inside himself some of her attentive holding. When he is clinging and holding himself together, he cannot take anything in, as that would involve stopping his holding-together activities.

As the mother and baby develop in their understanding of each other, this nipple-in-mouth holding function gets established in the mind and can be depended on more and more. The second-skin defences are resorted to less frequently or less desperately. The baby feels held together from inside. Then, for example, the baby is able to sleep through the night. Love between mother and baby is nipple-in-mouth holding. Perhaps what is called introjection is the establishment of this.

As the baby grows, these defences occur in a symbolic form— for example, the importance of routine, of the continuity in position of familiar objects, of memory to hold things in mind, and of intelligence to stick things together. The anxiety of spilling out or falling can be expressed in play and other forms of language, as can the relief of being found again and held. In children and adults, the unintegrated state can be expressed in a disturbance in thinking and communication as well as, on the motor side, in posture and mobility; in similar ways, so too can states of holding the self together—for example, a preoccupation with gymnastics may be to create a strong second skin.

Bick's theories are based on the idea of a body–mind continuum. She linked the concept of identity with that of feeling held together. This is a body–mind concept, and it is this that fluctuates moment by moment in the vicissitudes of infancy and motherhood. Her whole emphasis is on how the individual learns to survive in the face of catastrophic anxiety and, ultimately, to be able to contain it and to think about it. This ability depends on identification with or introjection of the containing function—that is, the nipple-in-mouth holding.

CHAPTER SEVEN

The relevance of infant and young-child observation in multidisciplinary assessments for the family courts

Biddy Youell

This chapter looks at the way in which observation is used by a multidisciplinary team in a specialist family centre, in which the central task is assessment and treatment of families with very young children where there are serious child-protection concerns. The cases are almost always in the court arena, and the team is employed as an "expert witness" in the proceedings. My purpose here is to demonstrate the way in which the team uses observation in its work and translates the understanding gained into evidence in written reports and cross-examination in court.

As a multidisciplinary team, we bring a wide variety of training experiences and theoretical frameworks to bear on our assessments of children and of their parents' capacities to care for them. Our most powerful tool, and the skill we have in common, is observation and the capacity to reflect together on what we observe.

I hope that the illustrations I have chosen will demonstrate how much we owe to the pioneering work of Esther Bick. It is a double indebtedness. First, what we are doing in family assessments and court work is a further application of the infant observation method that she introduced to the Tavistock child psychotherapy training in 1948. Second, our understanding of what we see is strongly supported by her thinking about primitive, infantile states described in her seminal papers in 1968 and 1986. The understanding of our observations of parent–infant interactions and of children's play is all too frequently in the realm of failures of containment, second-skin formation, and adhesive identification. I intend to highlight some of the features we commonly see in infants and young children and to make a link between them and the entrenched, internal structures that we encounter in their parents. The case examples I quote are some of the most distressing, illustrating, as they do, cross-generational manifestations of highly primitive, infantile functioning.

The task and the context

The task is to assess the parents' capacity to parent, and, where there has been abuse or failure to protect in the past, to assess their capacity to change. The team is asked to assess the children's development and to comment on any significant harm they have suffered as a result of their experiences. We are asked to describe the relationships between the children and each of their parents and between siblings. We are then required to make recommendations, itemizing the children's family placement needs, their educational needs, and their treatment needs, if any. If families are to be reunited, we are asked how to go about the rehabilitation; if they are to be separated, we are asked who should go where and with whom.

The team works from a shared belief that children should, if safe, be with their own parents. However, we no longer see this as the only positive outcome. Recommending that parents should not keep their children is never easy, but when we feel confident that we have done a fair and thorough assessment, there is some compensation in knowing that we have been instrumental in implementing planning for permanency early in a child's life. Repeated attempts to rehabilitate children may mean, in reality, that they are left in "drift" until they are suddenly deemed to be too old or too "damaged" for adoption. There are some babies who will have a good chance of a successful adoption because our agency, along with others, has faced the reality of what a parent can and cannot manage. Although they rarely see it as such, it is a good outcome for some mothers, who otherwise go on repeating abusive patterns of parenting.

Families attend the centre for one day a week over a five-week period. Each day consists of three clinical sessions, informal break times, and brief beginning and end-of-day meetings, attended by all staff and all families. The programme for each family is planned by the team, taking into account the background to the referral and the particular questions being asked in the "letter of instruction" from the commissioning authority. There are many differences between this kind of family centre and ordinary outpatient settings. The families occupy the space within the building for whole days. They have breaks between sessions, parents cook in the kitchen, children play up and down the hallway and in the garden. There are advantages and disadvantages. The building is small but well equipped, brightly painted and welcoming. Sharing facilities creates an atmosphere that most families find easier than the kind of professional distance and formality they associate with clinics. On the other hand, it means that there is very little privacy for anybody. They have to share the limited space with at least one other family, and parents are never left with their children without a member of staff being present. They know that even the volunteer workers, who are there to help them in break times, are making observations and that these may be used in the reports. While this kind of experience can, for some, feel like relentless persecution, it has been our experience that for most families it is seen as a genuine attempt on our part to get to know them thoroughly and to give them every chance to show their strengths. With the model of infant observation in mind, we try to help volunteer staff to achieve a benign, attentive, but non-intrusive stance when observing families.

Clinical sessions take various forms, with family members being seen in every possible combination. Children have individual sessions as well as taking part in parent-child sessions and full family meetings. Sibling groups are seen alongside parent or parental-couple sessions. Parents are seen by a key worker, who addresses the concerns very directly. They may also be seen by a psychiatrist for a psychiatric assessment, or by any member of the clinical team for a more open-ended exploration of their capacity to engage in therapeutic work. Some of the family sessions are observational; others are very clearly task-focused, within a systemic framework. In addition to the work at the centre, we make a home visit to children in the family home or in their foster placement. We talk to foster-carers, health visitors, and teachers, and, if appropriate, observe the children in school or nursery.

The work is discussed each week, and at the end of the five weeks we pool our experiences and our opinions and work together to reach a consensus. This usually involves vigorous discussions in which we may find ourselves in agreement or may find different team members holding very different positions. The team may be split, with one of us holding on to the concern about the child, while our colleagues may be in touch with something accessible and hopeful in the parent and may want to foster it. We are always aware of the dangers inherent in having rescue fantasies, based on the tiniest glimmers of hope, which all too easily disappear in the weeks between our involvement and the court hearing. Equally, we have to guard against an over-pessimistic, or even cynical, view that sees the cycles of abuse and deprivation as unbreakable. It is in these discussions that the multidisciplinary approach proves invaluable, providing, as it does, a system of checks and balances that we believe acts in the best interests of the families.

Observation

Observation has underpinned the training of child psychotherapists since Mrs Bick first introduced the method. Arguments in support of observational studies as part of other trainings are well developed (e.g. Trowell & Miles, 1991; Trowell & Rustin, 1991). Trowell (1999) has written about the potential for observational evidence to be used in assessments and in court reports.

There is agreement across the literature that attention to the countertransference is what distinguishes "psychoanalytic" observation from other forms of watching and recording human behaviour. It is this which we seek to metabolize in our multidisciplinary discussions and then to bring to life again in our descriptions of children in our written reports and when we give evidence in court. Of course, our evidence has to be presented against a backdrop of knowledge of child development, particularly when we are making assessments of infants and very young children. We need to back up what we are suggesting with knowledge of "the normal population" and evidence from outcome research in the field of family breakdown, adoption, and fostering. However, the power of the way we present evidence, when we get it right, is in the fact of it being so specific to the child or children concerned. Through using ordinary language and not shying away from emotional vocabulary, we show that we have engaged with the child's experience and know something about it. Even when the child is a very young baby, our infant observation training enables us to say something about the particular baby's individual response to his or her circumstances. Equally, we are, I believe, more ready than most "expert witnesses" to acknowledge what we do not know and cannot predict.

Assessment of children

One of the things that have preoccupied me in my role as child psychotherapist in the team is the discrepancy that often exists between our observations and the reports from other settings. The written notes usually focus on the positive aspects of the relationships between children and their parents. Contact sessions, unless actually disrupted by acting-out behaviour, are generally described in favourable terms. Similarly, the children are often described as "happy" or "contented" in their foster-care placements, as if nothing of the unusual and often traumatic circumstances of their lives has had any negative effect. The children who arrive at the centre with labels such as "independent, " "self reliant", and "undemanding" now attract particular attention from our team. We are alert to the fact that this so-called resilience may be indicative of a degree of withdrawal from intimate social relationships, which is seriously detrimental to their future development.

Clinicians trained in infant and young-child observation and who are familiar with Bick's notions of second-skin formation do not need to be told that a muscular toddler in perpetual motion is probably not simply "energetic and full of curiosity", to quote one report sent to us by a contact supervisor. Babies who are "calm" and "undemanding" are assumed to be "contented". There is often little awareness of the ordinary healthiness of a baby or young child who protests with vigour when uncomfortable and who is sometimes fractious and demanding.

To give an example: in a first encounter with one family at the centre, an 18-month-old boy busied himself, moving inexorably from one toy-box to another, showing absolutely no response to others in the room. He made no sound except for an occasional, expressionless grunt. His mother was alternately distressed and furiously angry with us and with the children. His sisters were sobbing. At one point, his mother got up, staggered across the room, and wrestled with one of the girls, who screamed. I, however, watching the scene unfold before me, felt astonished and deeply concerned that he did not look at his family, did not respond to the noise, did not make any approaches to them or to us for a whole hour. My colleague in the room was actively dealing with the events between Mother and her daughters, but I found myself detaching from the drama and focusing instead on the little boy's experience. In the countertransference, perhaps, I was understanding something of how he protected himself from unwelcome intrusion.

This child had arrived with the character sketch, "contented and delightful". Indeed, if we had videoed the boy in the session described above and somehow cut out all the other people, noise, and activity, it could have looked like a happy home-video of a contented child. When we wrote our report for court, we were able to recommend that plans for future placement should take into account his urgent need for a carer who would actively draw him into contact. We were able to describe his play and to illustrate his constant movement as he ranged around the room, but never stayed in any one place. He picked up and dropped toys at random, scarcely looking at them. We were able to show that although he smiled obligingly if spoken to and would allow himself to be lifted up and tickled without protest, he never initiated interactions and never minded when they came to an end; he would simply drift off and pick up another toy. He made no attempt to communicate vocally.

In another assessment, I observed a toddler, "Stacey", who moved around the centre like a small tank. She was the younger of two siblings, who, we had been told, were "unaffected by events". Their mother had almost certainly been responsible for extensive leg and rib fractures suffered by Stacey when she was a year old. Now aged 2, after a year in foster care she was described as "doing fine". I quote from an observation of her in a family session with her mother, maternal grandparents, and older sister.

Stacey stayed on the move throughout the hour-long session, approaching adults only when she needed help to reach the next toy that had caught her eye. She took possession of the space inside the playhouse and busied herself in activity with cups, saucers, and plastic food. Her play had a sterile, repetitive quality to it, as if she were simply doing what she had done a thousand times. Her grandmother remarked on her being a "good little housekeeper" and asked for a cup of tea, but Stacey did not respond. She was confident and well coordinated as she climbed onto the rocking-horse and rocked herself faster and faster, grinning exaggeratedly and gripping hard on the horse's head. I felt the excitement held her together and shut out everything else. Whenever her mother, her grandmother, or her sister approached her, she flapped at them frantically. Her voice was strangulated as she cried out, "Go away, no, no. Go away!" They laughed at her, telling me that she has always been like this, fiercely independent and self-sufficient. Standing close to her during one of these outbursts (and there were many), I felt a sense of absolute panic. Her entire body was vibrating with the strength of her terror at the threatened invasion. She held a pretend egg close to her chest, her fingers gripped tightly around it.

Her mother and grandmother then combined to get her to show off what seemed to be a kind of party trick. She was asked to repeat catch-phrases with appropriate accent and emphasis— e.g. "Bear with me a moment, please. Could you hold?" delivered in the voice of an over-cheerful telephonist. She completed her performance and then giggled obligingly; an anxious, shrill giggle. Everyone clapped. I suddenly realized that there had been no voluntary speech from her, other than her protestations that everyone should stay away.

Later in the session, she came close to me and I made a very quiet comment about the egg she was holding. She looked at me fleetingly before spinning off. She came back with more play food and dropped it in my lap. I thanked her. A few minutes later she suddenly sat at my feet and pressed her back against my shins with all her strength, as if getting as much surface-to-surface contact as possible. My feeling was that she was again finding a way to hold herself together and protect herself from intrusion.

In court, I talked about Stacey's behaviour and tried to establish some basic ideas to back up what I was saying. I was aware that I was speaking with some force in my determination to raise the level of anxiety about her emotional health. I talked about the fact that her imitative play was not imaginative or creative. I suggested that she could play independently but stressed the significance of what happened when an adult tried to join in. I reminded the court of the description of Stacey begging us all to "Go away". I suggested there was no sense of fun in her play and that the excitement she generated on the rocking horse seemed to be generated to avoid some other kind of feeling, perhaps terror. I further suggested that her well-developed speech was used not in the service of communication, but to maintain a manageable distance between herself and the adults.

We have come to think that there are many reasons for the discrepancy between what we read in reports and our own observations. Occasionally, an assessment has been done by a professional who has no experience of children, but this is not usually the case. The apparent minimization of the children's difficulties is more likely to be an unconscious response to the pain of facing what has really happened to them, and a defence against recognizing the degree of damage. In their paper on the value of observation in supervised contact, Hindle and Easton (1999) draw attention to the loneliness of the task for most workers and the tendency to detach in order to defend against being overwhelmed. Much has been written (e.g. Trowell & Rustin, 1991; Youell, 1999) about the function of the seminar group in containing the primitive anxiety generated by infant and young-child observation and its applications. In the family assessment centre, we have the un-doubted advantage, described above, of sharing the impact on us as individuals in a multidisciplinary team, which functions for us as a helpful container.

In addition, I believe that the discrepancy sometimes occurs because the children's presentation is genuinely confusing. These are children who have been repeatedly traumatized (whether through active maltreatment or through chronic neglect) from a very early age. Freud (1920g) describes a trauma as something that pierces the protective shield of the personality. The resilience of the individual in the face of the trauma depends on what has gone before. For many of the children we see in assessments, there is no "before the trauma". In Bick's terms, they do not have the experi-ence of being held together by the primal skin container, something she describes as being dependent on experience of an external object capable of fulfilling this function. The development of "sec-ond-skin" modes of functioning can then be seen as a "healthy" or perhaps "necessary" adaptation. Certainly, children like those de-scribed above have developed ways to protect themselves against intolerable physical and psychological intrusions. Their develop-ment is compromised, and there are interesting links between the kinds of behaviour we observe and what Meltzer (1975) describes as adhesive identification and which he links with autistic func-tioning. The "second-skin" phenomena we observe have much in common with autistic traits. We see children who smile with their mouths, in a defensive, muscular way, but whose eyes never smile. We see children who keep themselves company with strange, imi-tative vocalizations but who make no attempt to use words for communication. We see children who press themselves against hard, flat surfaces or who press surfaces or edges of toys together. We see children who point to a toy they cannot reach but who never point to achieve shared attention or enjoyment. We also see children who fit the kind of description that Bick (1986) gives of catastrophic anxiety of a fragmenting, liquefying, falling-into space experience.

Assessment of parents

Similar discrepancies occur between the descriptions of parents in the reports we read and the reality of our experiences when we talk with them and observe them with their children. We frequently see families where previous interventions have concentrated exclusively on behavioural techniques to teach parents basic child-care and parenting skills (nappy changing, feeding, etc.) and to encourage them to play with their children. This kind of work can, of course, be the first stage in establishing something much more lasting and meaningful in the parent–child relationship. Sadly, all too often we meet parents who have learned "the language" of child-centred play and who can talk about children's needs, for example, for routine and for boundaries. This kind of learning can mislead anxious professionals into believing that progress is being made and that there is real change for the better. Again, this is not conscious misunderstanding but is an entirely understandable, unconscious self-protection against the pain involved in reaching decisions about removing children and separating families. Sadly, the parents themselves can be equally misled by moments of rewarding interaction with their children, and it is often not until they are under pressure in an assessment such as ours, or later, during a monitored rehabilitation programme, that the imitative nature of the learning shows through and the two-dimensional structure collapses.

Bick (1986) writes "These problems of ego strength, two-dimensionality, adhesive identification and second-skin formation lie very deep in the unconscious and have their origin early in the preverbal period" (p. 70 herein). She goes on to suggest that patients with this kind of pathology require lengthy, painstaking containment before the underlying catastrophic anxiety will become available for scrutiny in the transference. Our brief work with parents in the family centre is different from long-term analytic work in almost every respect, but what we try to do in our limited time-frame follows something of the same track. We try to test out whether or not there is potential for change in the parents we meet, by seeing whether we can engage their interest in our way of trying to think about them. How do they respond to a thoughtful mind in a clinical session? Can we help them to be curious about themselves and about their children? Do our thoughts and words bounce off the surface, or do they find their way, at times, into a three-dimensional space, where reflection can occur? If they take on suggestions, do they do so in a merely imitative way, or is there evidence that the experiences might be becoming internalized? Does any reflective thinking go on in the sessions or, even more encouraging, between sessions? After some experience of our genuine attempts to offer containment, can the parent make links between their own painful and uncontained life experiences and those of their children, or can they at least make sense of the links we try to make with them? Do they allow us to have thoughts that they do not immediately discount or, alternatively, claim as their own? Words get incorporated into the script and are parroted back to us, with appropriate tone and emphasis but stripped of all meaning. As is the case with children, some deprived and traumatized adults somehow manage to hold on to something hopeful; some part of the personality remains open to an experience of containment. The preconception of a good object (nourished presumably by some actual, if minimal, good experience) has survived and is activated by the therapeutic exploration.

I shall illustrate the use of observational material in the court process more fully with reference to an assessment of a 10-month-old baby, "Kelly", and her mother. Kelly was the third child of Ms A. There were two older children from earlier partnerships. Ms A's current partner, Kelly's father, was a suspected paedophile. Ms A refused to leave him and the children were removed after the family doctor saw Kelly nearly at the point of death from starvation. Kelly was treated in hospital for five weeks before joining her half-brother and -sister in a placement with an experienced carer.

Before I return to questions about Kelly's development, I shall describe more about the assessment of her mother, Ms A. The links with the foregoing discussion of parental pathology are obvious. Ms A's history made disturbing reading. She was described as a shortsighted, unattractive, and overweight child of a single, deprived mother. Ms A reported that she was abused by an uncle and that she had become sexually active with peers at the age of 13. She said that they didn't seem to mind that she was fat and ugly. She had had several abortions and had given birth to three live babies.

Her partners were all sex offenders, and the older two children had
both been sexually abused at home.

It became clear during the assessment programme that the
driving force behind much of Ms A's life was an excessive interest
in and excitement about hospital treatments, medical matters, and
illness. Her talk was peppered with jargon from the medical
world, along with social-work phrases and the language of child-
protection procedures. Her barrister presented the fact that she
frequently took her children to the doctor and to Accident and
Emergency departments at all the local hospitals, as evidence of
her concern and protectiveness. Our conclusion was that it had
much more to do with her need to be a central figure in the drama
and to maintain a level of excitement. She was triumphant when
she told me that there was nothing she did not know about the way
paedophiles operate; I could rest assured that she would never be
"conned" into allowing one near her children.

With all this in mind, we tried to think about the meaning of her
having allowed her baby daughter to starve. We observed that she
avoided giving Kelly food or drink whenever possible, asking the
volunteer helpers to take over, so that she could "attend to the
older children". We asked her to take full responsibility for one
lunch with all three children while we observed. It was a hot day,
and she arrived almost an hour late because of taxi problems; she
was limping and pulling a shopping trolley. She was talking to
anybody who would listen about her damaged knee as her older
children came over to greet her. After giving them their lunch
boxes, containing huge amounts of sandwiches, crisps, yoghurt,
and biscuits, she took Kelly in her arms and put her in a sitting
position on the picnic table. Kelly had smiled when she first saw
her mother but now stared past her into the middle distance. Ms A
asked if the foster-carer had left Kelly's changing bag and com-
plained that she had spent a lot of money on it and had not had any
of the benefit herself. She asked if the foster-carer had left the
plastic spoon, and the next few minutes were taken up with her
complaining that there was no plastic spoon in the bag and finding
all sorts of reasons why it would be difficult to use anything else.

I was worried about Kelly's bare legs on the very hot wooden
surface, and another member of staff was asking if she had a sun

hat. Her mother opened a jar of savoury food and offered the baby a spoonful. Kelly was clearly uncomfortable, and she pushed the spoon away after two small mouthfuls. She waved her arms energetically and some of the food landed on her bib, some on the table, and some on her mother's teeshirt. She was red in the face and sweating but made no sound. Ms A insisted that Kelly had had enough and made as if to stop. I encouraged her to try again. She protested that Kelly did not like the flavours and said that she knew her baby better than I did; she was certain that the baby did not want the food. A few painful minutes later, I felt I had to tell her to move the baby into the shade. A volunteer helper organized a high-chair, and Kelly was immediately more comfortable and instantly very interested in the food. She ate hungrily from the spoon and looked eagerly at the jar. She finished it all. A little later, I suggested that she might like the pudding, but her mother insisted she had had enough and did not want it. Under pressure from me, she opened up the jar and gave Kelly a little, before saying again that the baby did not like it and trying instead to give her some of her brother's crisps. Ms A suddenly got up and left, saying she needed the toilet.

A week after the distressing scene described above, I tried to talk to Ms A about it. I said that I wanted to share an observation with her. I gently suggested that she seemed to have a real emotional difficulty about feeding Kelly. I told her what we had noticed and how it seemed to be the act of spoon-feeding or, perhaps, something about baby food which was so much more difficult for her than providing packaged food for the older children. She froze and then rushed from the room, choking, and shouted that I was making evil suggestions. She ran to the toilet and vomited.

When she returned a few minutes later, she was completely calm and told me at length about her tendency to throw up when under stress. All the shock and hatred had gone, and she was back in her familiar mode, presenting herself as the victim of yet another unusual medical condition. I could not find a way to help her to focus on what had caused the reaction, and she had managed to distance herself from it so effectively by this time that she was no longer seeing me as a persecutor. She was chatting to me again as if I were a neighbour at the kitchen table, a friend who would be bound to be impressed and sympathetic as she related more tales about her suffering.

By the end of the assessment period, we were faced with the inevitable conclusion that the children could not safely be returned to her, and that there was little scope for therapeutic work. There was no dissent in our team, nor in the wider professional network. Ms A's life was full of tragedy, and we felt a great deal of sympathy for her predicament, but we knew that her children would be at severe risk if they returned to her care. She could not make any use of our attempts to contain her. Here was a young woman who in Bick's (1968, 1986) and Klein's (e.g. 1946) terms was stuck in very primitive modes of functioning. She literally evacuated the entire experience of feeding and of what I talked to her about; she clearly experienced my words as a threat to her survival. I was left wondering about the links to her experiences of oral sexual abuse, but it was clearly impossible to explore any of this with her.

We were left with the difficult task of assessing the children's needs and presenting our recommendations in court. All of them were described as doing well in their foster placement. Each had their own story, but I shall focus here on Kelly, who, as mentioned above, was 10 months old at the time of our assessment. She attended the centre for three days with her siblings and her mother and was seen once at a contact session with her father.

I am quoting here not from our detailed observations in session notes, but from the condensed account, which went into our report. It is our practice to refer to staff by name in the reports (shortened to initials here).

> Kelly is a chubby baby with a ready smile. She reaches out to familiar adults, showing pleasure at the sight of both her mother and her foster-carer. When strangers speak to her in a friendly and interested way, she is quick to reward them with a smile. She also smiles at her siblings and watches them attentively if they are playing within her field of vision.

> The other side of this apparently open and cheerful disposition is a rather worrying absence of protest and a degree of self-sufficiency, which is not usual in a baby of this age. There were numerous occasions at the centre when one might have ex-

pected her to protest, to show her distress and to look for comfort from a familiar adult. She showed very little anxiety when
passed from her carer or her mother into the arms of a stranger,
and did not seem to register comings and goings. The one ex-
ception to this was in relation to her two siblings. She did seem
to be reassured by their presence and was markedly less settled
when they were out of sight.

There were occasions when she lost her balance or fell over but
she rarely cried. When she did so, she did not seek reassurance
and physical comfort, but turned instead to objects such as toys,
on which she focused until her distress subsided. This was very
apparent in the observation of contact with her father when she
repeatedly tumbled or banged her head and cried. She did not
look to him or to the other adults for help. When her father
lifted her on to his lap to comfort her, she arched away and
struggled to get back down on to the floor with the toys. A
similar sequence occurred in the session with J.G. after she had
bumped her head on a wooden bench. She allowed J.G. to scoop
her up and accepted the comfort for a moment, but was soon
indicating that she wanted to get away again and return to the
toys, picking up a plastic brick and pressing its edge against
her face.

There was some evidence of the beginning of language development in Kelly. If an adult made eye contact and smiled, she
would then engage in an interaction in which she tried to copy
sounds and rhythms. Her foster-carer confirmed that she was
doing this, and that she was sometimes heard to be babbling
when playing alone at home. She was also striving towards
being able to stand and greatly enjoyed supporting herself on
furniture. She was less keen on accepting the assistance of an
adult.

It is, of course, possible that Kelly's play was particularly repetitive and undeveloped in an individual session, where there
were no familiar adults and none of her siblings. However, the
same pattern was observed in other sessions. She spent long
periods of time sitting on her mother's lap, facing outwards,
and when put down with toys would bang them together or

push edges or surfaces into her mouth. She made no protest about being put down or passed from one person to another, and if a toy was out of reach she very quickly gave up and settled for something else.

The most alarming example of her lack of protest was in the family session, when her mother decided that she might be sleepy and put her down in the cot. She leant into the cot with Kelly in her arms and arranged the duvet as an extra mattress and then put the baby down in a way that made both workers feel very uneasy. She was allowed to drop the last couple of inches on to the duvet and was left there without any further talk, stroking, or reassurance. Ms A sat back in her chair and over her shoulder threw two soft juggling balls into the cot, with no regard for where they might land. Several times Ms A looked towards the workers for approval or in the hopes of their joining in a joke. It seemed that from the moment of letting go of her daughter she almost forgot her existence.

Kelly remained in the cot and made no sound but she did not settle at all. She moved around the cot relentlessly, pushing her face first into one side and then to the other. She pushed her head into the ends of the cot, rolled over, and turned around until she was almost spinning. S.S. commented later that she was reminded of an insect trapped and buzzing around. S.S. moved closer to the cot to look out for the baby's safety and Ms A appeared not to notice. After a few minutes, "Billy", her brother, climbed up and, stepping on a low stool, got into the cot, almost landing with both feet on his baby sister's head. Again, the worker was there, making sure that there was no harm done to the baby and helping Billy to manage as he climbed out of the cot. Ms A called out, "Billy! Out of there. Kelly's trying to sleep." It was patently clear that Kelly was not going to go to sleep and was becoming increasingly restless and uncomfortable, in constant motion, and almost doing headstands in her agitation. S.S. moved even closer and put her arm into the cot to protect the baby's head. Kelly seemed unaware of the proximity of the protective arm and continued to press her head into the cot mattress. Her face was red and shiny, with beads of sweat on her brows.

The above extract is an attempt to illustrate the way in which we incorporate observational material into written reports. We know that the lawyers and barristers will not read and digest too much detailed description; we therefore aim to bring the children's emotional life and internal-world experience to life in court so as to focus minds on their future placement and therapeutic needs. In the case of Kelly, the task in court was to convince the judge that she was not an ordinary 1-year-old, needing nothing more than ordinary care in an ordinary family. The damage in her two highly disturbed siblings was clear for all to see. However, the temptation in the network was to see Kelly, like Stacey, as too young to have suffered lasting harm. Much was made of her having reached developmental milestones, and her foster-carer described her as having a friendly and cheerful disposition, and a good appetite. We had to point out that her friendliness was indiscriminate and short-lived and that her lack of protest was not resilience but withdrawal. We described the desperate way in which we had seen her eat while at the centre, cramming food into her mouth and keeping an eye on her siblings lest they take what was hers.

In the witness-box, I was given the opportunity to talk in detail about the observation of Kelly in the cot and about the worrying nature of her silence and her turning towards comforting herself through contact with hard surfaces and edges. The judge wanted confirmation that she would not have suffered any lasting physical or psychological ill-effects from the starvation and was incredulous at the suggestion that her lack of protest might be a response to those early experiences. The judge was interested, but unconvinced, by the idea that children who do not get the response they need give up. She was, however, able to accept that in order to make the link between crying and getting the response they need, babies need to have hundreds of experiences of being attended to. She could see that Kelly had not had this experience and that her future carers would have to understand this and be prepared to provide these early building blocks of experience. With such persuasive observational evidence, I was able to talk about Kelly's urgent need for sensitive, non-intrusive, but *active* parenting to halt her withdrawal and, hopefully to bring her, step by step, into lively contact.

Conclusion

Training in Mrs Bick's infant observation method augments our capacity to recall the detail of what we see, to reflect on the meaning of our emotional responses, and to share our thoughts and feelings with those of colleagues. In cases such as those I have described in this chapter, her theoretical formulations give us a language with which to describe primitive psychosomatic functioning as well as to make some predictions about likely future pathology if appropriate care is not provided.

CHAPTER EIGHT

Mrs Bick's contribution to the understanding of severe feeding difficulties and pervasive refusal

Jeanne Magagna

This chapter examines the contribution of Mrs Bick to my understanding and technique of working with children suffering from severe feeding difficulties and pervasive refusal of life. During the most severe phase of their illness, pervasive-refusal children have their eyes shut and are unresponsive to pain or to any social stimuli. They are completely immobile and when lifted seem like a rag-doll, lacking a skeletal structure. They do not utter a sound, eat, drink, use the toilet, or care for themselves in any way (Lask et al., 1991). In "The Experience of the Skin in Early Object Relations" (1968), Mrs Bick describes primitive processes used to provide protection for the self fearing extinction. This is the starting point for my discussion of the pervasive-refusal child's use of "the blockading thumb". The metaphor of the blockading thumb is used because I view the human mind as an active agent: it seeks, in an active way, to create methods of protecting itself from what it perceives as a threat of annihilation. I do not believe anyone passively uses the primitive protections. Rather, I think that, even if it is deeply unconscious, there is at least some small element of active choice involved. The child, when completely alone and unprotected, has a choice—to stay with her [1] own emotional experience, the experience of something good, new, alive or something terrifying and bad, or to retreat and/or remain in a static "blockading-thumb" frame of mind. The blockading thumb consists at various times of the following five primitive processes: massive denial, bodily constriction and erotization, omniscience, omnipotence, and adherence to pathological parts of the self. The chapter also discusses how staff, the parents, and I incorporate Mrs Bick's method and understanding in the hospital programme for the children.

In some ways, the pervasive-refusal children are different from those described by Mrs Bick (1964, 1968, 1986). She focused on how, in a quest to maintain life and integration of the self, the infant uses various organs as suction pads. Eyes fasten on a light or the mother's eyes; the mouth sucks the thumb, holds on to the nipple after feeding; the ears latch on to the sound of mother's footsteps, the vacuum cleaner, or other sounds suggesting that family life is present. In each of these instances, the infant's organs, functioning as "suction pads", are reaching outwards to hold on to some object in order to cope with great anxieties of falling to pieces, disintegrating or liquefying, or dropping into a terrifying space full of "nameless dread" (Bion, 1962b).

In the severest phase of the illness, however, the pervasive-refusal child retreats completely—both psychically and physically—from contact with life. It is as though the soul of the self and perceptive organs have been completely barricaded against external life. The child loses ordinary mental functioning and memory. It is only in the process of recovery that the pervasive-refusal child's organs gradually function as suction pads latched on to external objects or events as a means of holding the self together and existing in the external world.

Examples of the blockading thumb

The observation of infants has provided examples of how retreat from the mother and the external world can ensue. When the trau-

---

[1] Feminine pronouns are used in this chapter since eight of the ten pervasive-refusal children with whom I worked were girls.

matized infant is not supported by the primary caregivers, the infant's method of survival ceases to involve the organs as suction pads latched on to external objects or events. Instead, there is a more enduring psychic and physical retreat. The following observation demonstrates an infant's temporary retreat using blockading primitive protections during the feeding time with his mother.

Example: Baby "Paulo", aged 3½ months. Mother anxiously holds baby, who is serious as he looks at his hand and rotates it in front of his eyes. Then with his left hand he grasps his right wrist and brings his fist to his mouth. Saliva bubbles are coming out of his mouth. Baby then sucks his tightly closed fist. For six or seven times, mother takes baby's hand from his mouth and baby returns it.

When mother shows baby the bottle, he looks at it as though he doesn't recognize it. He then turns away and looks at his rotating hand This is a regular pattern when the bottle is offered.

Mother pushes baby's hand away from his mouth and inserts the teat. Baby sucks once and spits out the teat. Each time this sequence is repeated, mother becomes increasingly insistent as she firmly presses the bottle hard into baby's mouth.

Baby grasps the bottle with both hands, pushes it away and spits out all the milk from his mouth. Mother becomes more nervy, intrusive, and angry as baby becomes increasingly strong-willed in wrenching the bottle out of his mouth, vomiting, and returning to sucking his fist.

Baby Paolo used his hand, fingers, and thumb to blockade access to his mouth and mind, which needed to be receptive to mother. However, since mother could not attune to his needs and contain his persecutory anxieties, he is attempting to use his thumb to find some security. He is feeling persecuted by the intrusion of the bad breast-mother. Mother is panicked because of her need to keep him alive. She is also angry and frustrated with her sense of impotence. By the end of the observation, baby, with his thumb in his mouth, seems to reside psychologically "inside mother" in a way in which he cannot be nourished by his external mother.

Similarly, the non-eating pervasive-refusal children are shielding themselves from life. They persistently retreat from a dependent position in relation to any person or from any experience that is felt to be intrusive. Here is an illustration of their retreat:

Example: "Cara", aged 9 years.   Eyes shut and body flaccid, Cara was wheeled through the hospital corridor towards the ward. She was emaciated and had a nasogastric tube, for she had been refusing food and drink for two and a half months. She seemed unaware of her urine-soaked clothing. Cara did not make the least perceptible sound or physical movement in response to noises, words, or touch. She remained motionless throughout day and night. She looked as though the cord attaching her to life had been severed. Her flowing, long, golden hair, serene and ashen face, and stillness gave the impression of an angel effigy adorning a grave. There seemed to be no emotional point to her existence.

Cara was one of ten pervasively refusing boys and girls, between 9 and 14 years of age, with whom I have worked in hospital. Originally the children had been placed in a hospital for non-organic pain, anorexia nervosa, or a virus. Hospitalization involved some separation from their parents, about which the children protested vehemently. They then gradually regressed into pervasive refusal of life and were referred to the hospital in which I work. When I first encountered these children, their loving link with their parents had been broken and they had given themselves up to death. This phenomena, called pervasive-refusal syndrome, requires psychiatric inpatient treatment for at least one year, followed by outpatient treatment.

The ten pervasive-refusal children's total immobility and unresponsiveness evoked intense anxiety in both their parents and the hospital staff. Having been deeply influenced by three years of infant observation supervised by Mrs Esther Bick, my work with these children and their caregivers was based on her way of understanding infantile emotions through using one's countertransference, while making very detailed, emotionally toned observations of the process of the child's nonverbal communication. Learning to make sense of their countertransference at each particular moment as a method of understanding the child's anxieties and use of primitive protections freed both the family and the staff to move from a sense of impotence, despair, and anger. They were able to observe, accept, and comprehend the children and in this way facilitate the children's movement towards life. Without any comprehension of Mrs Bick's notion of adhesive identification present in primitive protections, there was a tendency to intrude into the children's way of protecting themselves, to frighten them, and to force them into an even more fixed pervasive retreat from their caregivers.

Reasons for the blockading thumb of primitive protections

The human personality is like a mouth desperate for the mother's nipple to survive. We need personal intimacy with another to remain alive. For emotional survival, we also require intimacy between the adult and infantile parts of our personality. When either an internal or external trauma is experienced by a child, and the child does not receive sufficient containment to emotionally digest the experience, there is an attachment to the primitive protections. The blockading thumb of primitive protections prevents access to the mouth of the infantile mind hungry for love and understanding. The most important aspect of this blockading thumb is that the self must hang on to it to deal with the fear of disintegrating, falling to pieces, losing the sense of self and dying both physically and emotionally.

In the absence of an obvious potentially good "meeting point" with a protective, loving parent, this "blockading-thumb" frame of mind feels safe. Adhesion to the "blockading thumb" feels even safer than depending on the mother, who comes and goes. The timing of what appears to be "meaningless blockading" suggests an aim of plugging the mind with pleasurable comfort to avoid some experience perceived as meaningful and hence possibly threatening. Innate hopefulness, constitutional resilience, and environmental factors, including the capacity of the mother to provide primary maternal preoccupation, influence the child's capacity to bear distressing experiences. These factors are very significant in determining whether the child searches for a protective figure or turns away from humans to the blockading thumb of primitive protections.

Mismatched communication between mother and infant also influences the persistent, but sometimes almost invisible, use of the primitive protections in "a quiet baby". The "quiet baby" is denied the necessary nurturing, receptivity, and understanding the mother could possibly offer if the infant signalled her distress. The ten pervasive-refusal children's reputation as "quiet, good babies" may have been related to a barely visible use of the blockading thumb of primitive protections. Although in primary school the children seemed quite independent, in reality it seemed they were looking after themselves in a pseudo-mature way. Each mother regretted that although she wished to be closer to her child, the "child's style" was not to show many feelings directly or to confide much in her. For example, when questioned about experiences at school and various moods at home, the child often responded with "nothing happened", "can't remember", "don't know". It seemed that remembering and knowing would involve a basically un-contained child in feeling the threat of emotional significance that the mother would give to an event. One girl said she didn't confide in her mother because it would be distressing both to her and her mother.

The attachment to the "blockading thumb" of primitive protections rather than trust in her caregivers makes therapeutic work with the pervasively refusing child extremely difficult. Generally, twelve to eighteen months inpatient psychiatric treatment is required for recovery from being crippled by the symptoms of pervasive refusal, and then outpatient individual and family therapy is useful for at least one year.

In the course of treatment, typically the child begins to appreciate some of the external therapeutic figures. Then the child may begin to look at and listen more fully to these people. As the infantile emotions are freed and become more conscious, the child's dependency on the caregivers and attachment to the primitive protections can increase rather than decrease. Thus, psychological progress often alternates with retreat to primitive protections. This regression occurs at moments of misunderstanding, physical separation, or jealousy of others in relation to the person upon whom the child depends. The newly recognized infantile part of the child, no longer imprisoned by and dependent on the primitive protections, feels very thin-skinned and fragile. The child's terror, fear, and loving and hating emotions are excessive and frightening to her. Sometimes the intensity of her infantile emotions is also frightening to others. She cries, shows tantrums, or hits out, in a way that reveals her infantile emotions never consciously experienced or expressed when she was a baby.

When the child does not retreat to the blockading thumb of primitive protections, she becomes frantic, for she is not yet secure in her newly established dependence on the key external figures and she still lacks a resilient internal psychic structure to contain the intensity of her feelings. The child fears "disintegration", "falling to pieces", dissolving into a state of nothingness with no thing existing, no body, no self (Emanuel, 2001). She later verbalizes her terror of being pulled back into the prison of persistent pervasive refusal. Unable to bear the intensity of her newly emerging feelings associated with separation, frustration, misunderstanding, or jealousy, she feels helpless and occasionally once again "clings for dear life" on to the blockading thumb of primitive protections. However, now this retreat occurs for a few minutes, days, or weeks rather than for many months as is typical of pervasive refusal.

One essential question worth puzzling over is: what does the pervasive-refusal child do in relation to the external object at moments of conflict, misunderstanding, or separation? At first, there is no conscious hostility to the external figures upon whom she has depended. Why? Is she protecting a bond with a fragile, depressed object? Is she too afraid of reprisal by a harsh superego or punitive parent? Has the child unconsciously attacked the internal parents and damaged her developing internal capacity to contain emotion? Or has the fragility of adhesive, projective, or introjective identification to the external mother simply been disrupted in a way that the child simply fears falling into nonexistence?

When she could speak, one of the pervasive-refusal children said, "I dreamt I did not exist." Another said she dreamt that she was being shot. Each pervasive-refusal child may have unique and specific motivations for fearing non-existence and using each of the five common primitive protections. I shall now discuss each of these in turn.

The five primitive protections

Massive denial of reality

Cara, aged 9, whom I mentioned earlier in the chapter, was immobile, with her entire body huddled into a ball. A nasogastric
tube trailed out from under her hair, and this signalled her complete refusal of food which had occurred in her local hospital. She
did not make the least perceptible sound or physical movement
in response to words or touch. Cara's mind and body seemed to be
in a state of paralysis and disavowal of any sensation. She was like
a possum who remains completely still in a life-threatening situation.

A second child, "Rosa", aged 14 years, was admitted in a similar state. When she developed a normally extremely painful bowel
requiring an emergency operation, she gave no indication of physical pain either before or after surgery.

The lack of any response of these two girls suggests that they
were completely relying on massive denial as a method of blockading their awareness of physical pain and external impingements. If
they did have an internal response to pain, they were mute and
impotent in conveying their experience to anyone.

Massive denial was needed by the children when the world was
felt as totally persecutory. Paralysis, remaining completely unavailable, curled up, unresponsive, seemed to be the most basic
primitive protection against anxiety. It was hard to know if Cara
had a self present. At times it felt that only the bodily self remained
while the soul of the self had flown away.

Both girls seemed to be experiencing massive denial at times
involving a complete split of the conscious self from the body self
so that the body did not have any perceiving apparatus for mental
or physical pain. Whatever the mental state of the child, whether it
was disintegrated and not perceiving stimuli or that the conscious
self was completely split off from the body, there appeared to be
little if any opening of the mind for direct contact with the workers.

In a dream later reported by one of the girls, *her brain was
stuck inside a vase*. This suggested a mind that was blockaded from
experiencing meaningful relationships with others. Perhaps the
primitive protections are used to prevent the sane self from disintegrating, and, when they fail, the self falls into "the claustrum"

(Meltzer, 1992) represented by a brain being in a vase and barricaded from sane others. This same pervasive-refusal girl, after she had recovered, dreamt that *a monster came and poured liquid over her thus taking away all her features, her eyes, her mouth, her ears, her nose* . This dream reflected the girl's traumatic experience of no longer having access to the world through her senses.

It appeared that the two girls relied completely on massive denial as a "thumb to blockade" any response to internal physical pain as well as any external impingements. However, I knew from their histories that when they were not yet into pervasive refusal, both girls had vehemently protested when their parents left them in hospital.

Initially, Cara was in hospital for a painful mouth infection and Rosa was suffering from depression and anorexia nervosa. During their stay in their local hospitals, the girls gradually retreated into not eating and pervasive refusal of life. The girls' severe retreat to the blockading thumb of primitive protections—in particular, massive denial—seemed linked with having no containment for their physical and psychological trauma, which included separation from their parents and possibly not having the parents contain their own or the children's anxiety about the illness-promoting hospitalization.

When the girls started moving their bodies, they moaned and turned away from their parents as though, when the parents spoke or walked towards the girls, they were perceived as monster figures attacking the girls. The first picture that Cara drew in hospital was of a shark in the water. Her unconscious seemed to be like a sea in which only monsters were found. Cara's sense of persecution affected the various orifices of her body, including ears, eyes, mouth, and anus. Looking around seemed equated with discovering only attacking monsters, and gaze-avoidance seemed prominent for many months. Cara also later had dreams of being attacked by a monster and by a girl having razors coming out of her nails. She was always helpless and being tortured in her initial nightmares. Not eating, defecating, seeing, or apparently hearing gave the impression that Cara's soul had ceased to exist.

The question is, why did the girls choose to hold on to "massive denial" as a primitive protection? It seems that the girls' rage, directed towards the internal parental figures, destroyed the parents' goodness and capacity to function. The spaces both inside and outside the child's mind became frightening spaces. Lacking good and functioning internal parents, the girls perceived no possibility of having a good meeting point between themselves and another person. Life seemed pointless. The shark image in Cara's later drawing suggested that looking around was equated with discovering only attacking monsters, and hence the girls refused to look anywhere. Gaze-avoidance seemed prominent for many months.

Following several months of hospitalization, Cara responded to our approaches and talking by moaning as though she were being injected by a painful bite. Her first movements, some eight months into treatment, were crawling out of the therapy-room when she learned that her parents were going to spend more time with her on the unit. She had refused to see her parents for eight months, while idealizing the goodness of the workers and the safety of the ward. There was always a question as to whether or not the children's trauma and destructive phantasies were linked with emotional, physical, or sexual abuse or being bullied at school or at home. (Enquiries regarding this kind of trauma were not answered affirmatively except in the cases of two of the ten children. It was known that the father had used corporal punishment for Cara, her siblings, and her mother).

When later in treatment Cara's workers approached her, she responded as though she were receiving a blow, even though they were simply speaking to her or trying to lift her from the bed. Here we see how Cara's picture of her current world is distorted. We needed to ascertain if there was anything abusive or disturbing to Cara in her family environment. Certainly, in relation to hospital staff, Cara's distortion of her workers was formed through the projection of her frightening images on to them.

It was easier to understand when in response to a specific event a child gave a physical sign of retreat such as putting her hands over her eyes, physically curling up, holding her breath, or covering her ears. Through these signals of distress we learned how to modulate the immediacy, the emotional intensity, and the length and complexity of interpretations or communication of any sort. We also learned what upset the child and what was tolerable to her.

Gradually Cara more frequently peeped through her hands or hair and later glanced for a few moments towards the story being physically dramatized with the animals or dolls. When this occurred, the worker responded, acknowledging that there was a possibility of taking an interest in thinking about the story. What became clear over the course of time was how primarily following Cara's responses and giving them emotional meaning promoted a hunger for an emotional life with the key worker involved.

It was then possible for the worker to continue an interaction much like a mother does, describing all that she is doing to her baby while putting into words the emotional meaning of the physical expressions of the baby who is feeling very dependent and attached to her. Communication with the girls was used to alert the baby-self, enliven the baby-self, and make the baby-self a focus of attention (Alvarez, 1992).

Example. "You like that, don't you. You need to sit near me. When I go away you feel frightened without me to hold on to. You don't like it when I talk to someone else."

Through introjecting the experience of the key worker's following her state of mind, Cara was gradually able to feel that being emotionally connected to the nurse was good while being separated from her key nurse and being alone was terrifyingly bad. Cara was completely attached to nasogastric-tube feeding for a year. I understood this as her refusal to feed as a person separate from the feeding/understanding maternal figures. She seemed to be insisting on residing "inside mother" as though she had never sufficiently worked through the problems of introjecting a containing mother and separating from her. As a consequence, it seemed that an infantile part of Cara's personality was rather seriously split-off, blockaded through massive denial, and hence distant from her conscious, more pseudo-mature adult self. This is what Mrs Bick was describing in her discussion of the "second-skin", "carapace surface" hiding the unintegrated infantile parts of the self.

Through the containing presence of the hospital staff, alongside hospitalization involving separation from her mother, Cara became more conscious of and integrated her infantile feelings. This

introjection of a good mother, facilitated by the containment offered by her key workers, replaced an intrusive identification with
a pseudo-mature part of herself, consisting of the blockading
thumb of primitive protections.

The second primitive protection was used as the pervasive-
refusal child began to turn to the external world. This protection
was bodily constriction and/or bodily erotization, which I shall
now describe.

Bodily constriction and erotization

Joan Symington elaborates on Mrs Bick's thoughts as follows:

> the child's attempt to avoid the catastrophic fear of un-
> integration and spilling out into space and never being found
> and held again can lead the child towards tightening of the
> musculature. This involves a clenching together of particular
> muscle groups and maintaining them in this rigid position.
> This is an attempt physically to hold everything so tightly
> together that there can be no gap through which spilling could
> occur. It does not only occur with skeletal musculature but
> also with the smooth muscle of the internal organs so that the
> spasm might result, for example, in colic or constipation.
> [Symington, 1985, p. 481]

Responding to stimuli by stiffening and hardening of the
musculature represents the initiation of the pervasive-refusal
child's openness to the threat of annihilation in the outside world.
Stiffening of the musculature also represents a "struggle for survival", a struggle to live (Bick, 1968). Bodily constriction in response to negatively perceived stimuli was one of the first signs of
slight improvement of each of these ten children. Their bodily
constriction suggested that they now resided "outside the object"
and were freed to experience and respond, albeit fearfully, to the
world and begin the process of recovery.

For example, gradually Cara was able to find a self freed internally to respond to a frightening experience. She began recoiling
with tight musculature, closure of her eyes, and rigid posturing of

her hands and neck to stimuli of any sort. As her parents approached her, she would tighten her shoulder and neck muscles and bend into a ball, as though she feared being hit. When mention of going to the park was mentioned, she would again respond through rigid posturing of her neck and shoulders. At times, she would extend her fingers and hold them in this rigid position for a few minutes. A glance or a touch of a worker would be greeted as though it were a noxious impingement. Nothing seemed to be experienced as good. All these movements indicated that Cara was terrified of both external stimuli and her internal phantasies.

Two phenomena occurred at this point. First, Cara felt she had a self with a soul, and because she was more responsive to them, workers then found it easier to be involved with her. I became aware of how even an expression of pain or fear can be welcomed by the workers more warmly than the child's terrified immobility of all the senses. For several months, we usually experienced moments of despair as we faced the children's paralysed unresponsiveness to our efforts and came into contact with the child's inner experience of "giving up life".

> *Example.* When being asked to touch a cup of yoghurt with the tip of her finger, Cara recoiled with tight closure of her eyes, turning away of her entire body, rigid musculature in her tightly clenched hands. She also curled her feet, head, and body into the familiar fetal position of earlier days of her hospitalization. It now became difficult even to see anything but her back.

> *Example.* When she did begin to move, Cara also coiled herself into a tight ball, seemingly terrified by touch and by having any clothing taken off. The nurses often feared being abusive just in their efforts to change her clothes or comb her hair.

Second, self-erotization was clearly a protection turned to in the face of a bad experience.

> *Example.* When being wheeled down the corridor outside the inpatient unit, Cara responded by putting her fingers in front of her eyes and waving them about.

Example.   When she started to respond to her experiences by moving, Cara also began masturbating when alone at night.

Here we are able to see how Cara is now functioning in a different way. She has resumed the ability to differentiate between good and bad experiences. When frightened, good experiences are provided only through genital masturbation, the flickering of fingers before her eye, and tightening of her musculature to create a firm protection and hold herself together both physically and psychically. These actions function as a thumb blockading the mind from any experience perceived as bad and persecutory.

Primitive omniscience

Every step in development requires bearing the anxiety of a catastrophic change and an alteration in a sense of one's identity (Meltzer, 1986b). How do you navigate in a sea of terrifying objects? In her infant observation seminars, Mrs Bick suggested that you learn by watching very carefully, memorizing every little detail that signals the possibility of an impending disaster. You hold on to what you know, using it as a cue of what might happen in the future. You memorize details and facts and grip on to knowledge in a tenacious way, neglecting nothing. Omniscience is used as a blockading thumb in lieu of an internal container to bear the anxiety of sudden change. This primitive protection of omniscience demands mastery over details, a list of events, a schedule of what will happen and when. The mind seems a static space in which information is stored rather than a place in which thinking can take place. The known facts are adhered to rigidly. The baby-self requires that everything be understood in terms of whether or not it presents a danger to the self, which fears the terror of the unknown, falling apart, and dying (Bick, 1968).

The baby feels that there is no one, no mother, to pick her up if she does collapse, so she has to rely on herself, her own knowledge. It has to be omniscient, knowing everything. The omniscient self feels, "I must think and think I am so clever in order to protect myself." If the omniscient self admits that it does not know, the baby-self is lost, for it was dependent for its physical and emotional

safety on the omniscient self in lieu of an external or internal nurturing figure (see chapter 5).

Change and flexibility in an exploring mind brings the fear of
emotional issues, catastrophic anxieties, and imagination from the
infantile self. These threaten destruction of the fragile, more adult
part of the personality.

> *Example.*   The inpatient psychiatric-ward routine is structured
> and is therefore predictable.
>
> The pervasive-refusal children said that eating was even more
> difficult because they had lost the memory of the flavour of
> each of the foods.
>
> When Cara began to eat, she adamantly rejected any change in
> the eating plan. At first it simply seemed like a stubborn refusal
> to change from yoghurt to grapes, but gradually the nurses
> began to understand that Cara was still holding on to the same-
> ness and predictability of the routine meal of smooth vanilla
> yogurt with no bits and milk.

> *Example.*   A 4-year-old eating-disordered, neglected boy,
> "John", watched me each time I touched an object. He then
> incorporated each of my activities into his play. When I opened
> the door in a different way, or did anything out of the routine,
> he reminded me of "the right way to do it", which was to repeat
> the ritual of the past.

In examining knowledge acquisition of this abused boy John
and the academic work of these pervasive-refusal children, I became aware of how their schoolwork had a desperate quality, an
intense preoccupation with being rewarded by love and protection
from the teacher in order to evade internal fears. "If the teacher
doesn't award me the top position in the class, then who am I? I am
nobody, I am nowhere in the class." Any mark less than the top
mark feels like total failure.

There was no relief in having learned something, but there was
no intrinsic pleasure in any particular subject. Certainly, gripping
on to information was used to evade the uncertainty involved in
creative thinking involving the infantile emotions of love and hate.

Perhaps this is what led Einstein to postulate that imagination is more important than knowledge.

Primitive omnipotence

In the course of time, a growing child learns how to survive. The accounts by René Spitz about children dying in hospital if they were offered food but had no primary caretaker demonstrate how a child without an intimate attachment can die of overwhelming anxiety. The blockading thumb of primitive protections actually provides mechanisms to keep the child safe rather than dead from overwhelming emotional trauma. This is shown in studies of children raised by wolves, of those coming from severely abusive home situations, and those who have symptoms of pervasive refusal.

However, the massive use of primitive protections does not allow the child to develop. Massive denial, bodily constriction and erotization, omniscience, and omnipotence are used by the child to blockade the mind from the terrors—but also the beauty—of human intimacy. The infant part of the personality of a pervasive-refusal child makes a journey, which might be described like this:

Example.   "This feels terrible. What am I going to do? Turn away from it. Shut my eyes. Blockade my mind."

This is massive denial.

Example.   "This feels terrible, but my hands are good, they comfort me, that light in the ceiling is good, I can hold on to that. What I have to comfort myself is good. What comes from outside is frightening. Mummy comes and then walks away. This means I'm left in a sea of intense emotion with no point upon which to anchor myself except on good experiences I provide for myself through my play with my own hands, the light, and my bottom. My hands are good, they comfort me in front of my eyes. They give pleasure to my bottom. I can hold on to what I know, notice changes to.

"Avoid danger, hold on to facts so that I'll always know, never be no knowing. That provides security.

"I can only trust what comes from me, what I can do for myself. I must depend on myself. I can do everything for myself!"

This is primitive omnipotence. Using omnipotence, the self becomes idealized as a source of permanent comfort and "the other" becomes a recipient of all the destructive impulses. Gradually, there is an intense split between the self idealized as good and "the other" felt to be dangerous. "The other", however caring and thoughtful when approaching, now holds the destructive impulses that threaten to destroy the omnipotence of the self. For this reason, both caring and hostile human contact is viewed as being terrifying.

> *Example.*   What was striking about Cara and the other perva-
> sive-refusal children is how, when they started doing school-
> work and going to school, they needed to be encouraged to let
> go of their old habit of doing everything almost by themselves
> without support and without sharing any worries about the
> difficulties they were encountering. Cara wanted to keep her
> homework in her locker at school and share none of her difficul-
> ties about re-entering school after a year.

Adhesively adhering to pathological parts of the self

Underneath the common symptoms connected with pervasive refusal, each child had a different personality and pathology, which influenced her recovery process. Most difficult to treat were children who, as they began to come alive, in lieu of a healthy dependence on caregivers adhesively adhered to a malignant part of themselves that dictated orders to them. Three examples of this involve adherence to the dictating voice of hallucinations, a harsh superego, and the anorectic part. In all three instances, a destructive part of the self had been split off and was experienced almost as a separate personality. Gradually, the still fragile child began to depend on primary caregivers when they were physically present and in a one-to-one relationship with her. However, a problem arose when she had to share a primary caregiver or the primary caregiver was absent or was a disappointment to her. At these times, she adhered to one or more of these destructive parts of herself.

> *Example.*   One girl, "Maria", began to show more persistent psychotic features, including a hallucinatory big man who dictated that she was forbidden to either talk to the nurses or eat. She obeyed the hallucination for a long time.

> *Example.*   Another girl, "Annette", had a very harsh superego that persistently required that when she was alone in her room she should tear up her schoolwork because it was not perfect.

> *Example.*   A third child, "Sandra", had an anorectic voice dictating that she should starve herself.

Techniques of working
with primitive protections

I shall now explore some helpful therapeutic techniques that I developed in collaboration with parents and staff in working with these children.

The first message that parents and staff need to hear is a message that is hopeful and supportive of their wish to help the child. I say that although the child may not be able to eat, she is alive and is therefore still hungry for understanding; however, she is trapped by the blockading thumb of primitive protections in her ability to reach out towards them and towards life itself. I encourage respect and understanding of the fact that, lacking sufficient internal space for thinking about her emotional experience, the child feels that these primitive protections are essential for survival. If there is an attempt to take away the primitive protections too quickly and harshly, the child is likely to become distressed and terrified and will probably retreat even further from the caregivers. Therefore, it is important to share with the child the importance of these protections for her life, rather than to attempt to take them away. The parents also need to understand that the child is psychologically ill rather than simply "bad" in turning away from them.

The second message is to try to stop being intrusive—with force-feeding, by giving more than the minimum of necessary bodily care, by forcing the child to try to move, and or through asking many questions. The child simply needs to be clean, nourished, and sufficiently protected from others and from the cold. I suggest that we observe in detail both the child's physical and emotional state and our own moment-to-moment experiences with the child. We need truly to comprehend and contain the depth of the child's feeling, including terror and her severe anxiety in depending on us. I explain that if we understand our own feelings of being rejected, hurt, and frustrated by the child and feelings of being abusive to the child in doing ordinary care routines, we shall be freer to develop our capacities as receptive and loving figures.

The child will then introject our capacity of bearing emotions, and in identification with our healthy parental functions she will develop a psychological space suitable for bearing and thinking about her own emotional experiences. Once she feels profoundly understood and introjects the parents, the child will gradually feel less anxious to depend on her primary caregivers for support. This is because she will have internal parents to support her through the trials of separation, including what Bion referred to as nameless dread. Her newly developed internal psychological space, and her dependence on her external parents, will allow adhesive clinging to the blockading thumb of primitive protections to diminish in frequency and intensity. The child will then be free to consciously recognize and meet the needs of the previously obscured child-parts of her personality, which will emerge. When the child becomes more intimate with her own infantile emotions, there is a greater likelihood that she will also create more possibilities for her primary caregivers to understand that which worries her.

The third message is that the child will move towards health if we work very hard together as a team to be honestly receptive to our own emotional experiences in working together. The parents need to give the child permission to turn to the hospital staff and be close to them. We each need to use our countertransference responses to understanding both the child and the process of communication in the system comprised of the child and significant others. Unresolved conflicts, hostilities, and rivalries within the system working with the child tend to impede the sensitive child's development. In particular, staff members' criticizing rather than understanding the parents, and parents' jealousy of the staff, create difficulties for the child in relating to either group.

In terms of direct work with the child, the following ideas have been found to be useful. In the severest, immobile phase of pervasive refusal, when the child is using massive denial, the child fears being intruded upon with directly meaningful conversation. It seems more possible for the child to listen at first if the discussion is not about her, but rather about an animal. Even talking about "another person" seems too emotionally close at first. Because the child seems to have difficulty in staying focused on meaning coming from the therapist's words, using furry animal puppets and later small (3- or 4-inch) dolls seems to provide a pivotal point to gather and hold the focus of the child's attention directly to the child.

However, initially story-telling, using a puppet as the central character rather than the child, might still be experienced as intrusive if it is done directly in front of the child or with too much directness in telling "the story". It can also feel too intense if the theme is too concretely utilizing the child's current emotional experience. The fear of being intruded upon becomes obvious when the child will not show attentiveness when spoken to directly but will listen more readily and frequently if the therapist appears to be talking more to herself, to another animal puppet or worker, and to the side rather than directly to the child. If the child can freely choose to turn to or away from the drama, she is more likely to look and be attentive (Blake, 2001).

Story-telling was one of the most successful ways of communicating, because it was not intrusive and the child could investigate different levels of meaning within it. We described the story of "the little one" searching for protection by curling up, covering up, and staying still and away from us. We accepted the child's retreat as essential for the child to feel safe; however, we kept emphasizing that there is a search for safety. Later we described how one of the animals or dolls is finding different ways of searching for a safe place in his or her relationships. As the child fluctuates between attending and retreating from understanding, we would use the story-telling with puppets to highlight the dilemma of depending again on people or remaining linked to "the primitive protections" always available.

In summary, my impression is that the only way these ten children could be helped to release their attachment to the blockading thumb of omnipotence was through having a primary figure carefully following their emotional experience while giving meaning to their behaviour. A sequential process of interpreting seems to be useful in work with the infantile part. A useful progression seems to involve interpreting the child's need for security and the primitive protections, acknowledging the moment when interest and attachment to the key worker begins to develop, describing in detail the child's developing responses to negative experiences with the key worker and therapist, helping the child express panic and rage about feeling misunderstood or unsupported by the key worker and/or therapist, and accepting the love and dependence of the child. It is also important, when appropriate, to acknowledge the child's jealousy, possessiveness, and hostility to the other children. Such jealousy of others' importance to the staff provokes a different kind of dramatized, rather than emotionally intense, clinging on to the blockading thumb of primitive protections. However, more profound and influential in her development is a pervasive refusal's sense of loss of identity as a very ill child. This can contribute significantly to continued clinging to the primitive protections of pervasive refusal (Bick, 1968).

Conclusion

In this chapter I hope to have conveyed how there is an intrinsic meaning in every human activity and that one of the deepest human needs is to be understood in the context of an intimate relationship. Trauma, misunderstanding, and the lack of capacity to tolerate the separation from the mind of the other can lead to severe anxieties and use of the primitive protections. Criticism and pulling away the blockading thumb of primitive protections lead to more intense use of massive denial, bodily constriction and/or erotization, omniscience, omnipotence, and adherence to pathological parts of the self.

Mrs Bick's infant observation studies suggest that it is important to respect these blockading thumbs of primitive protection rather than intrude with too direct, too emotionally intense, interpretations directed to the patient. Mrs Bick's observational method using the countertransference accompanied by silent interpretations and verbalized understanding is essential to help the caregivers. It is her method that enables workers to consistently provide understanding to the deepest level of the pervasive-refusal child's barricaded infantile emotions. In this way, the child's anxieties about having a human meeting point can be mitigated.

CHAPTER NINE

Applying the observational method: observing organizations

R. D. Hinshelwood

E sther Bick developed the direct observation of the mother–baby couple as an aid to learning for trainees in child psychotherapy. This method soon produced research results, but Bick's primary aim was to accustom trainee child psychotherapists to the behaviour and inferred experience of the infant. During my own psychoanalytic training, I was fortunate to be in a supervision group with Esther Bick for my baby observation. I found myself enthralled by the depth of understanding that could come from the surface observations of the mother–baby couple and a profound insight into the process of unconscious interaction between the couple. It was not only this impressive depth, but the absorbing experience of being with a newborn and mother and, in my own way, "bonding" with them.

As a training experience, Esther Bick thought infant observation was:

> important for many reasons but, perhaps, mostly because it would help the students to conceive vividly the infantile experience of their child patients, so that when, for example, they started the treatment of a two-and-a-half-year-old child they

would get the feel of the baby that he was and from which he is not so far removed. It should also increase the student's understanding of the child's non-verbal behaviour and his play, as well as the behaviour of the child who neither speaks nor plays. Further, it should help the student when he interviews the mother and enable him to understand better her account of the child's history. It would also give each student a unique opportunity to observe the development of an infant more or less from birth, in his home setting and in his relation to his immediate family, and thus to find out for himself how these relations emerge and develop. In addition he would be able to compare and contrast his observations with those of his fellow students in the weekly seminars. [Bick, 1964, p. 37 herein]

I took from this that her purposes were

- to conceive infantile experience;
- to understand nonverbal behaviour;
- to become more familiar with relations with parents;
- to contextualize development, and how relations emerge;
- to compare and contrast the observation with those of fellow students in seminars.

Psychiatric trainees

As a consultant psychotherapist in a large mental hospital back in the early 1980s, I too was confronted with a training task. My job, in part, was to try to interest young psychiatric trainees in psychodynamic thinking. Could I make psychoanalysis sufficiently engaging? Would it be useful for their future work? Would they *see* it as sufficiently useful? When I came to consider this task, I recalled the observation course in my own training and began to wonder about an observation experience for them.

Though the psychiatric trainees were bright, they were stuck in a culture that induced in them a scientific attitude to their work and to the objects of their study, the patients.

The psychiatric context is notoriously difficult for psychoanalysis and psychotherapy. Freud remarked in 1916:

Psychiatry does not employ the technical methods of psycho-analysis; it omits to make any inferences from the *content* of the delusion, and, in pointing to heredity, it gives us a very general and remote aetiology instead of indicating first the more spe-cial and proximate causes. But is there a contradiction, an op-position in this? Is it not rather a case of one supplementing the other? [Freud, 1916–17, p. 254]

Since then, with the extraordinary power of medical science, scien-tific psychiatry has evolved even more to view the patient as a distanced object of study and less as a suffering person (Hinshel-wood, 1999). My task was to make the suffering person as relevant as the scientific object of study.

Infant observation
and psychiatric training

I rejected my initial thought that they could engage in a compara-ble infant-observation, because I thought that it would not *feel* relevant to psychiatric trainees. What, I asked myself, was the equivalent of the infant for my trainees? What did *they* need to conceive of vividly? The first thought was the psychotic patient, but I had considerable doubts about trainees, not in analysis them-selves, being able to confront psychotic patients with the necessary calm attention. The focus of infant observation is, in any case, a relationship—that between mother and baby—and I wondered if trainees might observe something equivalent in the ward: the rela-tionships between those working and those residing there. If infant observation was a step to learning to conduct a therapy or an analysis, could ward observation be a step to learning how to lead a psychiatric team on the ward? This placed the observation in the arena of psychiatric culture and of the relational dynamics of that micro-society.

Infant observation and the social system

If I was to use the observational method, it had to be transposed to a social and cultural context, and this is problematic for an individual psychology such as psychoanalysis. However, a long time ago Malinowski wrote in a somewhat critical article that he thought that Freud had nevertheless given the basis for the genesis of social institutions:

> Freud's contribution to anthropology is of the greatest importance and seems to me to strike a very rich vein, which must be followed up. For Freud has given us the first concrete theory about the relation between instinctive life and social institutions. [Malinowski, 1923, p. 650]

Whereas in infant observation it is the relationship between mother and infant that is observed, in a social setting it is the attitudes of interacting groups that must be observed. In fact, there have been psychoanalytically inspired investigations of this kind (Obholzer & Roberts, 1994; Trist & Murray, 1990). The most well-known at the time that I was beginning (in 1982) was the classic study by Isabel Menzies (1959) of the nursing service in a general medical hospital.

Menzies study was based on Jaques's (1953, 1955) theoretical exposition of the concept of the *social defence system*. It was not an observational method but one based on questionnaires and interviewing. However, the results gave a paradigm for understanding the insertion of the individuals, unconsciously, into the collective phenomena of the social group. Regarding the individual, she wrote "the objective situation confronting the nurse bears a striking resemblance to the phantasy situations that exist in every individual in the deepest and most primitive levels of the mind" (Menzies, 1959, p. 440).

These phantasy situations in the individual mind, because they are shared (or there is a good deal of overlap between individual nurses), transform into collective phenomena. Following Trist (1950), I understood that the psychoanalytic approach must focus on aspects of the *culture* of a group as it interacts with other groups with their own specific cultures.[1] In fact, Trist's original conception

---

[1] This theoretical framework, as well as the observational method, is elaborated in Hinshelwood and Skogstad (2000).

of culture was that it bridged between the unconscious of the individuals and the social phenomena. Important aspects of culture could be perceived as collective unconscious phantasies, expressed as defensive aspects and assumptions in a social group. Menzies' description of the nursing service addressed unconscious attitudes to the work they do that nurses held and reinforced in each other. These cultural attitudes are based on extreme phantasy situations, which are conceived in quasi-magical terms. The phantasies concern the violent damage that nurses believe they have inflicted on their patients and then the omnipotent restoration demanded of the nurses. These phantasy situations are not consciously shared, since these phantasies are unconscious. Nevertheless, they influence conscious thinking and can be observed in the way the nursing tasks are actually practised. The unconscious phantasies are realized and reified in the specific nursing techniques that are used and, in fact, taught to students.

The social defence system of a nursing service

Menzies described a number of practices that seemed to solve problems that arise from the level of the unconscious situation, rather than the actual problems of the working tasks. One instance is the "task list" system. This meant that a nurse would go around the ward performing a single task on each patient—taking the bedpan to each one, or taking the temperature of each one. The result was that no nurse related fully to a patient, but only to a "part" of each patient—the excretory function, or the temperature, and so on. It looked to Menzies as if this kind of practice was driven by unconscious sources. The depersonalization of patients protected nurses against the experience of damage and the demand for magical cures. However, it seemed to arouse frustration and disaster for the nurses themselves since, consciously, they felt the lack of personal relations with their patient, wanting both the satisfaction of helping another human being and the eventual gratitude of that patient. Thus the patient seemed to become a depersonalized object, and this frustrated nurses in their motivation to help people.

Anxiety/defence in infant observation

Menzies' study relied on the psychoanalytic model of anxiety and defence. This, too, is fundamental to Bick's observational method, which also rests on the basic psychoanalytic proposition of anxiety and defence. Bick noted the anxiety of the mother, who is beset by concerns about her adequacy; at the most basic level, her body functioning (her approach to labour in the first instance and, subsequently, baby-care—lactation, for example) and also her ability to handle the infant, protecting it from too much distress. Mothers engaged in many different practices to evade these concerns, which in turn often interfered with the "maternal reverie" (Bion, 1962b) or "primary maternal preoccupation" (Winnicott, 1960).

Bick was even more interested in the experience of the baby. Increasingly she concluded that the primary anxiety of the baby was a fear of falling to bits, or indeed on occasions when help was not available, the actual experience of leaking, dissolving, liquefying—a spaceman in outer space without a spacesuit was one of her preferred analogies. The baby has to cope with this experience in various ways—particularly prominent among which were the various forms of "second skin"—and eventually she evolved her theory of adhesive identification. She evolved an extensive theory of skin sensation and of its crucial role in giving the baby the sense of having a boundary, something that gave the baby the sense of holding together.

In relation to my training task, I thought that the levels of ego function were quite different with young adults. So the key idea I took from both Bick and from Menzies was the psychoanalytic anxiety/defence model. For Bick, it was the falling-apart anxiety and second-skin defences; for Menzies, it was the anxieties of care and the defensive techniques of the social defence system. There was, in my view, therefore, a considerable correspondence at a theoretical level, close to the observed level that could inform the details of the observational material in both cases. In other words, I thought that there was a correspondence in the psychoanalytic approach to both forms of applied psychoanalytic observation.

In addition, my aim corresponded exactly with Bick's. It was to sensitize the psychiatric trainee to human relations, anxiety, and defensiveness, just as hers was to sensitize future psychotherapists, and analysts, to the infant's relationships and to their anxieties and the ensuing defensiveness. The object of infant observation was that the observer should be sufficiently part of the family to feel the emotional currents as they occurred and then (or subsequently) to think about those emotional experiences.[2] My observational intentions were also for my trainees to be sufficiently close to the emotional currents of a ward and then (or subsequently) to be able to think about those experiences.

This is a psychoanalytic stance—to be able to have an experience and to be able to think about it at the same time. This is what I wanted to help my trainees to achieve, to the degree that each one was capable. They were deeply immersed in a culture made up of a set of social attitudes and value systems, which they adopted at work unthinkingly, about patients, treatments, and staff–patient relations. However, to be better psychiatrists I believed they needed to think about their culture and to understand some of these currents of emotional attitudes and values into which they are inducted by joining the profession. In helping to sensitize my trainees, I wanted them to concentrate on this form of subjective observation, which Bick's method seemed to offer. The sets of attitudes and values of the staff team, when confronting their patients, could be discerned from the trainees' human response to being on the ward, just as the observer of a mother and baby makes observations as much on his or her emotional response to the mother's handling and the baby's responding.

---

[2] Entering the family in this emotional way prompts unconscious anxieties that are well known to psychoanalysis—notably, the oedipal experiences that emerge from witnessing a couple in intimate relationship. Britton (1989) described the problem of the Oedipus complex as the task of achieving a "third position", one that is not in identification with either partner of the couple, but witnessing the intercourse from an excluded position. Insofar as a mother's baby represents the fruitful intercourse between mother and father, the observer is required to achieve a witnessing position from outside that parental couple. Observation is thus an opportunity to revisit these issues, and a further chance for working-through. The observation is a developmental opportunity and thus, to a degree, an adjunct to the observer's own analysis. Seminar leaders need to bear this potential set of oedipal issues in mind for all the members of their group.

Observation has two strands: one is the objective performance of the tasks and any striking conflicts with the task; the other is the emotional response to what is happening—in the case of psychiatry, the interplay between the attitudes of the psychiatric service and their patients. Furthermore, a psychoanalytic paradigm would contribute an understanding of the hardly owned, or unconscious, aspects of these attitudes.

Thus, my method involved attending to the behavioural practices of staff, just as Menzies had observed and recorded the defensive practices of the nursing service. By inference, she then related such practices to individual defences in each nurse, defences that are supported by the social system of attitudes and values. This method corresponds exactly to the observation of mother's behaviour with a baby. In both cases, the inferential aspects of the method—moving from observed behaviour to postulated underlying anxieties and defences—is informed by the emotional experiencing of the observer.

Examples from a ward observation

I shall take as an example of ward observation that reported by Donati (1989). She was, in fact, the first of the trainees to undertake an observation as a registrar in psychiatry. She observed a typical "back-ward" from the old-style mental hospitals and conducted it in 1982. There was a characteristic form of interpersonal contact.

(a) *The observed behaviour* is described thus:

Throughout the sessions while I was just sitting in an armchair, looking around, my contact with patients was largely restricted to exchanges of smiles and looks. The patients very rarely spoke to others; this was not because of gross cognitive impairment as there were some who could play cards, chess, draughts, snooker extremely well, frequently beating the nurses!

Both patients and staff would break this isolation in two ways: (a) on their way in or out of the ward ("Is it time for TO?", "How was the walk?", "Why don't you go out for a coffee?", "How are you feeling today?"); and (b) in brief comments to the various passers-by who were captured momentarily with a challenging, appreciative or jokey comment from patients who were sitting in armchairs as if waiting for something to happen. This *touch and go* behaviour involved everybody. . . .

I have illustrated how the patients made feeble attempts but failed to make contact with me, and how staff responded to this. On two other occasions they tried again: the first involved a patient who usually walked up and down:

"Are you Dr V's secretary?" — "Why?" — "Just to know." — "Do you need to see her?" — "Not really." . . . "What nationality are you?" — "Have a guess." — "Welsh?" — "No, have another one." — "No, I give up." When he came back he insisted on knowing my nationality. He then said a few words in Italian so I asked: "Have you been to Italy?" — "Yes, during the war." — "As our rescuer?" — "I don't know about that . . ." And he left.

This seemed another example of the *touch and go* behaviour and the difficulty of establishing genuine and deeper relationships. [Donati, 1989, pp. 37–38]

The defensive techniques were clear and persistent. It was a method of reducing personal contact and, thus, the anxiety-provoking phantasies of damage and restoration. This was supported by a stereotyping of patients into men and women and the consequent moulding of the nurses' role:

I was received by the patients without question as to who I was and what I was doing there with them. Beneath the superficial impression of being accepted lay doubt about the real degree of personal contact. I was put, after all, in the same position as the patients and the general quality of the relationship seemed more of a depersonalised and stereotyped kind:

The nurses came back and went on chatting about "how much better the female chronic wards are since women are capable of making wards their home, they are always doing something, looking after themselves and their environment. The atmosphere is much more alive, cleaner . . . more at home. Male patients neglect themselves, need continuous encouragement, find the place boring and the nurses have to try to make the ward like a home . [p. 36]

It was also was reflected at lunchtime:

At 12 o'clock sharp the dining-room was full, the music very noisy. The charge nurses dished out the meal. A staff nurse took it to the

patients. The patients mostly ate without exchanging words. They
were distributed at the tables according to different "types". One was
the table of the overeaters (obese-diabetics) who "needed to be checked
and who should not eat from each other's plates". Another was the
table of the poor eaters. At a single table a blind patient had food
placed in front of him. The other two tables were occupied by mixed,
more balanced personalities. [p. 41]

As can be seen from this, at meals patients were ordered according
to their specific feeding characteristics.

(b) *The felt experience* of the observer was characteristically similar to what she had observed with the patients. This excessive
ordering gave the ward a lifeless atmosphere, impersonal and
over-managed. She described how a particular nurse needed to
feed her too:

This was the first of his several forced feeding moves towards
me and the patients. He wanted repeatedly to feed me with
coffee, milk, biscuits, fried chips, etc. Although I tried to convince him that I wasn't hungry he wouldn't believe me. Perhaps he had projected on to me his own sense of deprivation in
the ward starved of life, and was defending himself against the
loss of his nursing role. He was feeling I was hungry, thirsty
and was impelled to feed me. [p. 39]

The impact on the observer was powerful—"forced", she called it.
And she tried to understand the pressure of the nurses' anxiety to
perform a visibly competent role. Her sense is that the nurses
found themselves in a chronic ward where many aspects led to a
pessimism about their ability to do much for their patients. She
intuited that they felt "impotent" and then needed to respond to
that in some way so that the feeling could be discharged. She was
very alive to the despair that threatened these male nurses.

Was I less threatening if seen as a female visitor, object of
masculine comments, instead of being seen as a doctor visiting
their ward with the possible view of discovering their life?
    I left feeling surprised about the unexpectedly rich material
and emotional experiences observed during the hour, and at
the same time worried and guilty. [p. 35]

The observer's experience was uncomfortable in this ward, as she
sensed that she might be threatening as a doctor who would look

into their ward and, presumably, discover things that they might not want exposed.

(c) *Inferences* can be made from this dual material of observed behaviour and felt experience. In considering the arrangement of the tables at lunchtime, she brings together the behaviour—the depersonalizing over-orderliness—with her experience—being perceived as a threat—and makes a deeper analysis of the emotional structure of this little society:

> This organised sub-grouping prompts some questions. What is this need for order, control and management in a setting where the staff complained about boredom, lack of initiative and co-operation amongst the patients, and about the draining dependency? How are unexpected happenings viewed? Do the staff promote activity, co-operation, personal initiative in the patients?
>
> It seemed to me that, in response to the experience of failure and impotence in nursing chronic patients, there arises a defensive urge to extinguish any sign of spontaneity, involvement, emotionality and expectations and to keep everything lifeless, predictable so as to avert new hopes, new disappointments and intensified frustration. [p. 41]

Thus, the anxiety about impotence generated such a control that it had to extinguish spontaneity, which might become threatening. However, the lifelessness itself generated a renewed feeling of impotence. As Donati pointed out:

> There is a *self-perpetuating cycle* in all this: Threat (of impotence, loss of identity and skills, fear of outbreak of mad, sexual or aggressive excitement) arouses anxiety, leading to ineffective defensive manoeuvres which increase the threat and thereby the anxiety. [p. 43]

In a ward devoted to containing, controlling, and treating chronic madness, it is not surprising that anxiety about mad outbursts is a daily threat. The problem here is that the response to such a threat—a sustained lifeless culture on the ward—is maladaptive, feeding into the fear of impotence at enhancing a truly better quality of life for their indefinitely prolonged charges.

There is here a persisting anxiety that suffused the work of the staff and the life of the patients. This anxiety arose from the feeling of impotence, a lack of support for professional skills, the uncertain identity of male nurses, and perhaps above all the "madness" of patients, which could catastrophically challenge any sense of potency, skills, and identity. In response, specific defensive techniques were embedded in the work practices. These comprised the maintenance of stereotyped and depersonalized relationships, expressed most obviously in the touch-and-go behaviour; a rejection of the staff's feelings of impotence and despair, by projecting those feelings into the patients; and the extinguishing of any sign of spontaneous life, and emotional relatedness.

The culture of the ward therefore appeared to express attitudes that embodied both an anxiety about madness and the fear of coping with it, and a defensiveness against those anxieties. This describes the interplay between the unconscious anxiety of the individuals, and the collectivization of defences in the sets of group attitudes and values which result in work practices. Thus the observation is not just the way people work, but the meaning that behaviour has in terms of work anxieties and relationships. What I realized the trainees were observing was the collective intra-group attitudes, and their expression in inter-group behaviour in the highly stressful work of a psychiatric team. In applying an observational method, I was in the event heartened that I could in fact tap into the "humanity" of the trainees and find them very willing to think about the relationship of care.

Sensitizing the trainee

Initially each trainee was supervised by me, individually. However, I soon began seeing three or four in a seminar, as in Bick's observation method. The trainees initially assumed that the life on typical psychiatric wards was dead, but they became enthused by my encouragement to see if there was more "going on" than met the eye. We wanted to know if there was an "underlife", as Goffman (1961) called it, and whether that could be understood in terms of the psychoanalytic unconscious. Initially, for me as well as for them, these were questions we were jointly investigating. As the project progressed, trainees became interested in specific questions, such as about what happens in an acute ward, or what life is like in a social services after-care hostel.

The presentation by the trainees of their records to colleagues in a seminar adds an important dimension. Through the unappreciated aspects of the observer's presentation of his or her record of a session, the seminar can help him or her to sharpen subjective experiences into a new instrument for understanding the human situation he or she is surrounded by. In the observer's written process records and verbal asides when presenting to the seminar, the observer presents a pesonal account of his or her own sensitivity—conscious and unconscious. Turns of phrase, particular emphases on certain events or people, particular asides (and often those proffered with a humour that seems to dismiss them), and so on are very important to pick up on. A weekly seminar will acknowledge the tensions and support the trainee. However, it is a receiving apparatus for the conscious and unconscious sensitivity.

It is impelling for these observers' learning that each has personally made the record in which others see things he or she has not seen. They can then reflect and assess for themselves whether this feels true and, if it does, they can only grant that it was spotted by themselves even though they might not have consciously registered it. Again and again, naïve observers have found themselves impressed and excited by how much they have retrieved of their experience in a setting that has often seemed in advance to be characterized by its dullness or deadness. For instance, one observer, who in fact chose a class in a sixth-form college, [3] was presenting material about the dilatoriness of the young students in doing some task set by the teacher. The observer then conveyed to the seminar, as an aside, something about the future life for such students. The seminar picked up on the aside and began to discuss the sense of responsibility for future lives that is felt by teachers and the school. This could then be formulated as a specific anxiety of that educational setting, for which specific defensive techniques (connected with discipline, perhaps) may be established. This dis-

---

[3] The observation method has recently been taken up by professions other than psychiatry and in settings other than health care.

cussion led the trainee to convey a good deal of surprise and an appreciation of the insight.

Conclusions

I want to review the five bullet points with which I started:

- to conceive infantile experience;
- to understand nonverbal behaviour;
- to become more familiar with relations with parents;
- to contextualize development, and how relations emerge;
- to compare and contrast the observation with those of fellow students in seminars.

In this observation method evolved for psychiatric trainees, there are corresponding aims:

1. to provide the experience of the anxiety in the system;
2. to understand that the behaviour at a cultural level is similarly nonverbal;
3. to become more familiar in a sensitive way to the attitudes and values of the staff team as they relate to their patients;
4. to understand how these unspoken and therefore unchanging relations develop from the anxieties and collective need to defend against them;
5. to use the seminar as a tool for supporting and probing the unconscious of the trainees and their unconscious understanding.

The potential is that trainees can retain more composure in the staff teams and with the colleagues with whom they work.

My initial question—whether psychoanalysis could be made interesting and relevant to psychiatric trainees—seemed answered satisfactorily.

The capacity to take an objective view of the problematic relations between psychiatry and psychotherapy and to "feel" the experiences of this is a dual skill. It is, moreover, a skill that is the fundamental form of practice of modern-day psychoanalysis. Thus, there is a psychoanalytic quality about the use of the results of this method. Insofar as this is not psychoanalysis, because the setting is quite different, there is nevertheless a psychoanalytic quality about the dual stance that is in use. In fact, it is quite possible to use the psychoanalytic terms "transference" and "countertransference" for some of the phenomena—and indeed this is often encountered. In defence of the psychoanalytic nature of this project, we can consider Freud's "psychoanalysis" of Little Hans, and of Judge Schreber. Both these "cases" of Freud's dispensed with the psychoanalytic setting. In the first it was Hans's father who conducted the discussions with the little patient. And in the case of Judge Schreber, Freud confined his analysis to the published memoirs of the judge.

In Bick's observational method, the observation was of the relations between a couple, a couple of which the observer was not a part. In the present project, this is true but their relations are of inter-group relations—those between the group of patients and the staff (mostly nursing staff). Thus, I would claim that the method does give a psychoanalytic insight into a field that is not psychoanalytic but is one of social science. The method is potentially a practical contribution to social science as much as it is to a training method in psychiatry.

CHAPTER TEN

Secondary skin and culture: reflections on some aspects of teaching Traveller children

Jan Dollery, with Andrew Briggs

I n my work as a teacher for children of an Irish Traveller community, I [J.D.] have benefited enormously from being part of a regional observational course, associated with the Child and Family Department of Tavistock Clinic. Through seminar discussions, I have begun to develop a deeper emotional understanding of my encounters with the children and their families. This growing awareness of the setting in which I work has begun to help me see things about the community that I was not so aware of previously.

For those interested in or working with Travellers, our understanding of their culture has advanced through the pioneering work of the social anthropologist Judith Okley (1983). Her study was the product of a three-year participant observation of a Traveller community. In this chapter, I discuss my provisional thoughts about Traveller culture from a different perspective. I have begun to see more clearly that not only is individual behaviour determined by cultural beliefs, which is part of Okley's thesis, but that these act as a skin-like external container for the individual when an internal container, already extremely fragile, is ineffective. Although by no means clear at the moment, what is emerging through my observations and encounters with children and families is cultural beliefs acting akin to what Mrs Bick in her seminal papers (1968, 1986) referred to as a substitute container for terrifying infantile anxieties. Furthermore, this container also acts as a determinant of parental attitudes and practices, through which the reality of a fragile internal container is reproduced transgenerationally. Within this backdrop, apart from allowing me access to such an important and little understood culture, my work as a teacher has enabled me to be of some emotional assistance to the children and their families of this community.

The Irish Traveller community

The material for this chapter is drawn from my contact with, mainly, one extended family. Irish Traveller families are part of a wider Traveller community that includes Gypsies, showmen from fairs and circuses, New Travellers, and bargees (canal-boat dwellers). Irish Travellers belong to a distinct ethnic group, which differs from the Gypsies observed by Okley in terms of historical background and geographical origins. There are, however, similarities in their cultural traditions. In highlighting aspects of Okley's work on Gypsies, this forms a starting point for suggestions about the Irish Traveller community.

Okley recognizes that the culture is an attempt to retain a social identity. Here she recognizes that certain cultural beliefs enable maintenance of the "symbolic boundaries". These are necessary because Gypsies are "under constant pressure from the dominant society to become assimilated" (1983, p. 77). Okley also recognizes that the Gypsies see "culture contact" as potentially bringing about change "by a kind of contagion" (p. 77). Thus there is a daily pressure on individuals to remain separate and different from the dominant society. Furthermore, under such duress, group integrity "must be maintained and expressed in some independent way" (p. 77). One way of remaining different is through pollution beliefs, which, Okley says, "express and reinforce an ethnic boundary" (p. 77). She continues:

The complex pollution taboos indicate that the Gypsies can be said to make a fundamental distinction between the inside of the body and the outside. The outer body symbolises the public self or role as presented to the Gorgio. The outer body or public self is a protective covering for the inside, which must be kept pure and inviolate. The inner body symbolises the secret ethnic self, sustained individually and reaffirmed by the solidarity of the Gypsy group. [p. 80]

Women are not allowed to bring certain parts of their bodies into contact with a man, except during sexual intercourse (strictly defined as within a marital relationship). The wife's underwear has to be washed and dried separately from her husband's, and out of his and the community's sight. If a man inadvertently sees a woman relieving herself, this is a pollution of him. Breast-feeding has to be done in privacy. Indeed, Okley notes, "I found that the vast majority of women avoided breast-feeding altogether and opted for bottle-feeding, despite the contrary advice of midwives and health visitors" (p. 208). Since defloration of wives on wedding nights is also seen as a loss of purity and, therefore, potentially polluting the husband, it is not surprising that menstruation is seen in similar terms. Okley records some cases of wives not being allowed to cook during menses. Also, specific mention of menstruation in front of men is not allowed. When she came across examples of some families not seeing menstruation as dangerous pollution, she found that "childbirth always seems so" (p. 211), both being "occasions for the outlet of body waste" (p. 211). Furthermore:

> The baby is ambiguous matter because it has been covered by the blood and waste of birth: the inside come outside. The baby remains polluting for a while, possibly because it has not been "made" a Gypsy until some socialisation has taken place. [p. 211]

In the dominant culture, sexuality, childbirth, and child–rearing are all things that, to a greater rather than lesser extent, evoke (usually) pleasurable emotions for those involved. The fact that Travellers carry taboos about these, reinforced as powerful cultural beliefs, indicates a terror of emotion taking over the individuals and threatening group solidarity. This solidarity—what might be termed a social skin—is driven by the fear of pollution by the dominant culture. In this, the fear of pollution would suggest that the culture and individuals exist in what Klein (1946) termed the paranoid-schizoid position, as contagion appears to be equated with persecution. But such persecutory anxiety does not stop here. The worry about what comes out of a woman's body suggests that there is a more immediate sense of the world inside the culture being a polluting, contagious, one. With this as the cultural and individual mindset, there are serious repercussions on the growth and development of individuals, parents, and children. From an educational stance, the main one is the development of the child's curiosity and its effects on academic and social capacities. I want to turn now to discuss these consequences, in the light of what I understand to be a cultural lack of capacity to think about emotions in a sustained way.

Culture and thinking

When speaking to Travellers on their own territory, there is initially a sense of relating to differing individuals with strong personal characteristics. However, over a period of time, it becomes evident that the lack of individual growth and development leads in many cases to members of the community seeming "to develop the social appearances of a personality but without any real sense of an inner mental space and internal resources" (Miller et al., 1989). Without this sense of individual inner strength, Meltzer (1974) argues, a more "two-dimensional surface relationship" to objects evolves, one where imitation and copying of the other takes precedence over internal principles that have been generated by internalized relationships. He describes this process as "adhesive identification". In this, I would argue, Traveller culture provides a framework to which individuals can adhere, be given an identity, and feel held together. Age-related separations that might lead the individual to be aware of a lack of internal substance do not occur. For example, the children remain with the nuclear family until they marry, and therefore they never have to survive the experience of being physically alone and outside the extended family.

The community acts and responds in a very concrete way. The culture not only encompasses physical movement from one place to another, but also a continual mental shift away from stimuli that might otherwise evoke difficult thoughts and feelings. On site, the Travellers visit from one trailer to the other. Cars ferry people to and fro. Off site, in church services or the cinema, there is a constant movement in and out of the building and a hopping from seat to seat, person to person. The relentlessness of this movement is an example of the individual's use of the defence of "second skin" as described by Bick. The physical use of the body moving from one stimulus to another seems to hold the individual together in an almost sensual way and denies the possibility of there being a prolonged space in which to think. This defence, however, is ruptured at times through acts of violence, within both the family and the wider community. These lead to disruption and disperse the family, causing it to collapse and fragment. Eventually the families coalesce again when they return to the site. However, because emotions cannot be held on to and processed, are dealt with through constant activity, or are evacuated, often through acts of violence, there seems to be a perpetual, non-evolving, repetitive, cycle in which a status quo is maintained. This is the order of things that exists when there is no capacity to reflect upon the underlying issues, and no digesting of events that can provide links that might later be recalled and used productively in a similar event.

The constant activity one can witness on and off the site is part of the culture's expectation of individuals. By being part of it, individuals bind themselves together as individuals and, hence, to the culture. This is how their social skin, functioning like a secondary skin, keeps formed. In this, individual membership of the group brings them the opportunity for what Miller describes as the "rudimentary parts of their personality [being] somehow made to cohere" (Miller et al., 1989). However, as Bick's discussions of the children she treated make painfully clear, secondary skin is a highly fragile formation to protect an extremely fragile, almost non-existent, ego. Hence, it is not surprising that powerful emotional events are defined and bound by taboos. However, it is also clear that these taboos are themselves fragile, and this not more so than for the ones concerning the inside of the body, especially of the woman's body. This was made clear during the following incident, which most graphically demonstrates Okley's observations of the polluting potential of what comes out of a woman's body. I am using this as an illustration of second-skin functioning and the puncturing of this.

A young mother, having given birth by Caesarean section, was naturally horrified to witness her stitches come undone in the trailer. Her husband and family, she said, had seen "her insides hanging out". The family had run around screaming hysterically. While the family were obviously concerned about her physical health, I think the event resonated at another, deeper, level. Her split skin divulged a space that exposed inside parts that were too terrible to witness, perhaps a concrete representation of what is feared will overwhelm if activity ceases. The mother spoke of how the sight of her insides had made it difficult for her husband to be attracted to her. While this might have been due to the taboo about her body the fact that she later became depressed suggests that the belief system as a skin was holed for her, and she found poor containment through trying to hold on to it. On one occasion when I visited, she had just let down all the tyres of her van. They were now as depressed as she was and rendered useless in offering an opportunity for escape. In this way, she ensured that she remained tied to the site, attached to the culture in a very concrete way. Hence, she remained with those who shared her fear of disintegration, which further reminded them, as her spilling out had done, of their own vulnerability.

This incident throws into focus a number of related themes. First, it is clear that the sight of the woman's insides filled her husband with something like what Bion (1962a, 1962b) referred to as "nameless dread". Obviously terrified by being suddenly persecuted through his wife's insides coming out, he could not differentiate his feeling of falling to bits from the sight of her actually spilling out. In this he may have felt, as Mrs Bick described for extreme cases of disintegration, that he was becoming liquid. He certainly appeared undefended, like one of Mrs Bick's illustrations, an astronaut without a spacesuit. The cultural beliefs he held on to, the process that had acted to protect him, now left him naked in outer space. Another aspect of this incident is also associated with thinking. This man's beliefs had been inculcated into him since childhood. Later in this chapter, the consequences of the taboos concerning the woman's body as antithetical to emotional, and its link to cognitive, development will be explored. For the moment, however, one might hazard a speculation and say that, had his development included curiosity about his mother's body and that curiosity had then been helpfully contained by her, his capacity to think about this event in his marriage might have been stronger. This, however, and as already stated, is not a question about individual container–contained relationships as such, but more an observation of the pervasive effect of the culture on them. This culture is one in which taboos prevent curiosity taking form, as it is a culture where a thinking space is discouraged through the taboos acting as a harness on the self, and as an attempt to ensure that that which is split off and projected remains so.

For children raised within a culture that operates, for the most part, in the paranoid-schizoid position, splitting off from consciousness certain experiences and feelings, it is likely that the capacity for symbolic thought will be greatly impaired. To some extent, this is discussed in the following section. Because the children's development has been affected in this way, I have used a very concrete teaching style to help them decode the symbols of written language. This is discussed later in the chapter.

Child development

Sexuality being taboo, it would seem that its outcome, pregnancy, is likewise. Some women tell me of how they knew nothing of menstruation and had only a hazy idea of what was going to happen on their wedding night. Granny recently informed me her youngest daughter was going to have a baby. I asked how far on she was in the pregnancy? Granny looked startled, lowered her eyes in embarrassment, and said she did not know. So, even before the birth occurs, it is hard to imagine the kind of mental space a pregnant mother might be able to give to the baby growing within her bodily skin. However, such restricted thinking being around before the birth seems a likely contributor to the mother's limited capacity for sustained thought for her newborn baby. Tender moments between mothers and their babies are witnessed during feeding, as the child is held securely in their gaze. The babies, however, are universally bottle-fed, enabling the care to be shared with the eldest daughter or other members of the family. The baby is encouraged to grow up quickly. A mother quite firmly tapped the cheek of a 12-week-old baby I had been given to hold and declared, "We've told her she is a big girl now and there is to be no more petting!" When a few months old, it is common practice to see a baby left lying with a bottle propped near it, an object to fix on to in the absence of its mother. This attitude to childcare may be a way of sparing the parents having to experience the vulnerable infantile bits of themselves—that is, as a defence against intense feelings of envy, jealousy, love, or hate evoked by the presence of their baby. One can understand that, with no strong internal parent of their own to contain these infantile responses, they may be felt to be unmanageable. However, they are also examples of a reproductive process for the limited containing object. With these comes the reproduction of difficulties in withstanding primitive infantile feelings. So, because the parents have difficulty bearing their own primitive infantile feelings, they cannot adequately contain the primitive infantile projections of their babies. Because the parents do not adequately contain these, the baby is left with them. Mother provides for baby an object to be stuck on to, but not one that can be penetrated by curiosity and known from the inside. When discussing the epistemophilic instinct, Klein (1923) highlighted learning disturbances if the child's curiosity about the insides of his mother's body is curtailed by her inability to recognize this. Later, Bion (1962b) added the importance of the K link. A mother unable to link with her infant, through trying to understand his experiences and feelings, may be introjected as an object that does not have the capacity to think. In the more extreme circumstances discussed here, introjection is also of an object that is fragile. All this stunts the growth of the infant's personality. As the material and discussion of this chapter show, the processes bringing about this stunting are within the interpersonal relationship of mother and baby but are also a function of the culture.

Despite their suspicions of the dominant culture and its agencies, by and large Traveller parents appear very keen for the children to acquire the literacy skills they do not have, and they are supportive of primary education. However, OFSTED (1996) reports show significant underachievement of Gypsy and Irish Traveller children from the age of 7 years onwards, in relation to age-related national expectations. It is difficult to know what happens between the early years and age 7 to bring about such a dramatic underachievement. Certainly, the children from the extended family I am drawing my examples from have immense problems in learning to read and write. Many parents, however, see secondary education and the mixing of teenage boys and girls away from the site as a threat to their strongly held moral values. They fear also that their children will be introduced to drugs. Many see prolonged schooling as an impediment to maturity and think that, after the age of 11 years, the children should be working alongside their parents—the girls learning how to keep family and home together, while the boys are initiated into the family trade. Apart from these, more instrumental, reasons why children may be picking up messages from parents about how far to go with their education, the latter may fear they will lose their children if they became too identified with the settled population. What I am beginning to recognize, however, is that children's sticking to culture allows no space between it and them; feelings are concretely felt but not considered, for they are sealed by the tightness of the fitting together of the surfaces. This culture is one where persecution outside is feared. Aggression from within is managed by adherence to culture and cultural identity, but it is not processed. When the social skin is punctured, there is, for long moments, nothing to hold the individual together, as personal secondary skin is so bound up with the culture. From my observations, this internal situation is acquired very early in a child's life. Hence, like that of their forebears, the internal situation is one where persecutory anxiety is enormous and only just contained by a pseudo-skin.

That this intergenerational reproduction of the culture's incapacity for sustained thought is unchecked by anyone from within the culture might suggest that the concept of childhood, as a period of vulnerability and growth, is not in the parental and cultural mindset. However, there are times when one can see that children are very securely held in mind, as adults do have immense   concern. These examples of something like containment of the children's feelings by adults come to the fore when a severely dramatic incident almost punches the cultural belief system, to elicit a response through the a hole. Such responses lead me to believe that it is not so much an *absence* of containment but, rather, a limited one. This is seen in the following example:

> A few months ago, Granny took into her home her youngest son and his children; a girl aged 18 months and a boy 6 months old. Their mother had committed suicide shortly before Christmas. Soon afterwards, father received a custodial sentence. His daughter's distress was clearly understood by the family, as was her relief once she had been able to visit her father. Granny frequently states that she thinks it will have a detrimental effect on the child when she grows up, but there seems to be no hope expressed that anything might be done to change or lessen the prospect. She recognizes the importance of answering truthfully the questions asked by the child, but she finds it difficult to bear the distressing accompanying emotions. She understands the baby's need to hold on to her as he drifts into sleep and remain pressed against her through the night, but she does not talk through this need with him. One aunt told me about the jealous feelings between her niece and daughter as they fought for her attention in bed one night. She resolved this by sticking one child on her chest and another in the crook of her arm.

The incidents show that the adults recognize that the children are in pain, which resonates within them. However, for reasons already outlined, the feelings are then quickly denied and the response is to provide for the children a sticking of a skin-to-skin form of containment. Nonetheless, *I suggest that this experience of being held in mind is securely internalized by the children and provides for them a limited source of internal support during difficult times.* Because the whole process is fraught with fragility, the underlying emotions remain unprocessed, and this has a detrimental effect on the development of thinking processes within the individual child.

Teaching Traveller children

I want to start by mentioning two examples that have helped me see my role as teacher far more clearly.

I once asked an 11-year-old girl what it meant to her to be a Traveller. Without a moment's hesitation she replied: "Everything." There was no space in her thinking between the word Traveller and herself, no sense of her as an individual belonging to a culture. What she seemed to be expressing was an equivalence between self and the Traveller cultural heritage. This close, sticking to, relationship between children and culture has profound consequences not only for their social development, but for their educational development too. I often observe the muscular way in which the little girl mentioned above, now nearly 3, conducts herself around the site. She frequently pushes and occasionally drops a bike that is much too big for her to ride, but to which she appears desperately attached. In the absence of an internalized consistent object to hold herself together, she seems to have adopted a "pseudo-independence", as she walks alone from one trailer to the other with the bike. This mode of second-skin functioning serves to contain her for some of the time. However, it proves too difficult to sustain indefinitely, and, when it deserts her, she drops the bike and is left floundering in a state of distress. At such times, there appears to be nothing left inside to support her once the skin-type holding collapses, although it is evident that painful feelings continue to be felt internally. She then anxiously attaches herself to any adult relative present, repeatedly asking of them, "Do you love me?" The reassurance she is given brings only temporary relief. She veers from a pseudo-independence to being adhesively dependent on the concrete presence of an external object. When a family member is not available, and especially if a child is away from the site and its culture, I am the one used in this way. That there is still hope in the child of finding an animate, real, object for help with feelings suggests that there is a thought that a container exists, even if the concept is that it is something to stick to. Perhaps this little girl's plea "Do you love me?" carries the concept that something good can be felt inside if something good is taken in from outside. It is, in other words, a concept of containment. It may be pushing the material too far to suggest that she has in mind a full concept of an internalized containing object, as described by Bion (1962b). Bion discussed the importance of a particular state of mind in mother, a "maternal reverie", which is receptive to her child's primitive emotional communications. This involves her not only registering her baby's primitive emotional communications, but also being able to tolerate and think about them long enough to then return them in a transformed state. Through this her baby's development is established. This attention and support for the infant's state of mind, her capacity to withstand, process, and digest his feelings of anxiety and fear of falling apart, creates a relationship in which her mind acts as a container for the baby. Bion referred to this dynamic and complex interaction as the container–contained. The baby is then able to introject the feelings in a more modified and manageable form. Miller summarizes this as its becoming "the source of a rudimentary trust in himself and his surroundings which allows the baby to relinquish his mother's external presence and enables him to begin to turn instead to internalised images of her" (Miller et al., 1989, p. 29).

My contact with these two girls helped me to become more sensitive to two aspects of my role. The first is as a facilitator for the children's transition from Traveller to the settled community's culture found in the nursery or school. Salzberger-Wittenberg (1983) describes this as "a delicate transition, helping the child to extend his relationship from within the family to those with teachers and with children of the same age group". The second is directly as a teacher. Here, I have become more aware of the need to think on an emotional level about academic tasks.

Although the children are aware that I do not belong to their group, through my presence on site and my relationship with their families I provide a concrete link for them, a reminder of something perceived of as safe and familiar in an otherwise alien world. My relationship with the children often starts before they are three years old, which allows trust to be built between us, in preparation for me transporting them to nursery. This first trip to a formal educational setting is recognized as an important step by the parents, possibly as a sign of the child growing up and is often talked about with the child for some months before. Frequently, several family members will be present to wave the child off when the day finally dawns. When on site, the children sometimes follow me around, which seems to be an indication of their need to feel held and contained. They recognize in me a capacity, difficult though it is at times, to bear witness to the knowledge of events that befall them and an ability to put into words feelings that they are unable to express. When with the children, I sense that it is important I affirm their demonstrations of affection, which may be mocked at home by some family members as a defence against painful feelings of intimacy. I offer praise whenever possible to bolster self-esteem. To engender trust, I am stringent about carrying through what I have said I will do. (Sometimes at home, the children are told untruths to pacify them or to control behaviour.) Most importantly, I try to promote emotional literacy by making space and time to help them think about, and name, feelings that are often put into me or are acted upon instinctively and immediately. Klein (1932) noted the emotional importance of a child being able to make use of language to the full extent of its capacity. Britton (1998b) writes that "the word provides a container for the emotional experience, putting a semantic boundary around it". Very often, I am left feeling disturbed as the children relate, in a matter-of-fact tone of voice, incidents of violence they have witnessed. At such times I usually make the comment, "that must have been very frightening for you to see", which is sometimes confirmed but frequently denied. Two more specific examples where words are containing are as follows.

For a long time, Granny's young ward would try to climb into my car, saying, "Me nursery Mrs Dowy." Several times a week, I would repeat that she was too little now but that I could take her to nursery when she was 3. There are times however, when words cannot be taken in. She would continue to fight her way inside, and when putting her out again I was left to experience her acute feelings of longing and loss. I deliberately tried to provide a containment similar to that of her culture by chanting the same words each time, as if it were a mantra, in the hope they would provide something for her to fix onto. She eventually began approaching my car with an appreciable difference. Then she started the sentence "Me can come to nursery", and I replied, "Yes, when you are three and a bigger girl." She would nod, and I would leave without feeling a wrench. It seems to me that only after first being held together by the words could she then take them in and make sense of them. This was successful because, along with the mantra, I was a live object that she could use and internalize.

An example where words said by me contain the child's feelings and go on to develop a containing dialogue is found in a later stage of my work with a young boy, "Miley".

Miley started school at the age of 4 years. Within an hour, he had been told off by the Head for climbing on chairs and tearing up the class register. Living and sleeping as he did in close quarters with his siblings, I felt it was difficult for Miley to know where he ended and others began. He would continually interfere with his classmates, hitting, pulling, biting, strangling, and rolling around the floor with them. To deflect any thinking about this behaviour, he would run away from the protesting adults and spit at them when they tried to talk to him.

During one barrage of spit I said, "Miley, babies spit because they can't talk, some animals spit because they can't talk. You *can* talk, so stop spitting and tell what is wrong." The spitting stopped. Verbalization took longer. Each time I was with him and observed him acting out (e.g. shouting out "   BASTARD" throughout a song because unusually he had not been chosen for a role in it) we talked about the feelings of not being chosen that were being expelled. By being a supportive adult female, I often represented mother for him. He would act out his feelings of need for his mum with me. He did this in a way that was not possible with her, for fear of being ridiculed by his elder siblings. Thus he would run up to me and clasp his arms around me, making it difficult for me to tear myself away. He would lay his head on my knee during registration and hold on to my hand throughout story time. He became possessive of me, not wanting my time to be shared. This sticking to me felt like a powerful experience of adhesion, as if he had stuck to my skin. One day I heard him say twice, when trying to find space to sit on the carpet and then a place in a queue, "there's no room for

me", perhaps symbolizing his feelings of being pushed off his
mother's emotional lap and replaced in mind by his younger
siblings.

Two months after starting school, I supported him in a PE
lesson. Afterwards a group of children surrounded me and
asked for help with shoes. I heard Miley shout, "Mrs Dollery."
I turned and said I would be with him in a minute but then saw
the class teacher approach him to offer help. A few minutes
later, he came up to me, holding his shoes. I smiled at him. He
drew back his arm and punched me straight in the eye. It hurt,
and I felt shocked, tearful, and angry. Through this attack, he
managed to communicate to me his anger, arising from painful
feelings of longing and envy. He resented the many children
with me who prevented him from having sole possession, like
his siblings did with his mother. When I had recovered, it was
clear to me that his striking me was his only response, because
he was unable to process feelings, as he had nothing inside to
help him do so. I took Miley into the hall for a private talk. I
explained that he had hurt me and asked him why he did it. He
replied, "Because you put the other's shoes on and not mine." I
said, "You were angry because I was helping the others instead
of you. What could you have done instead of hitting me?" Miley
was unable to reply. I said, "You could have said, 'I'm very
cross with you Mrs Dollery. You are helping the other children
and you're not helping me!' And what do you think I would
have said then?" Miley answered, "Yes." The following week, I
made a green caterpillar to help him learn the colour green. He
wanted to take it home. I explained we needed to use it the next
day but then he could have it. Five minutes later, Miley said to
me, "I'm very cross with you Mrs Dollery." I said he was a
clever boy to be able to tell me that, and I explained that I was
worried that it would get lost in the trailer. Another five minutes passed and he said, "I'm still cross with you." We discussed the matter further, and Miley agreed to wait until the
next day for his caterpillar. Being able to move a step further
and *think* about a solution to his problems took longer. Just
before Christmas, Miley's cousin, "Michelle Ann", started
school. I found her weeping in the playground and decided to

take her in to meet her teacher before the bell rang. Miley, who up until then had been playing happily with some friends, wanted to come in too. I explained that, unlike him, she did not have any friends in the playground and was feeling lonely. He thought about this for a moment and then announced, "I know—I can look through the window", which he did for several minutes before running off to play.

Conclusion

In this chapter, I have given a brief outline of my contact with an Irish Traveller community and tried to show how particular cultural beliefs shape attitudes to childcare and development. I have argued that such beliefs are in the service of denying the opportunity to think about emotional life. Such is the extent of this denial that culture can be seen to act as a social skin, in the manner of secondary skin formation described so closely by Mrs Bick. This skin holds together the individual within the culture of the community. Without this skin, there would be a sense of individual and collective terror in the face of unprocessed thoughts and emotions pouring into the private and public domains. The individual examples I have discussed show the resilience of this culture but also that it punctures when something dramatic hits it head on. Through examples of my contact with children, I have recognized that there is hope for a more reflective emotional engagement, and that this is possible through helping them feel safe enough to find the words to describe their experiences. What I am doing with the children is, for the most part, the antithesis of their experiences at home. In this, I am mindful that my hope to help them develop an internal container places them in a difficult position between two cultures.

CHAPTER ELEVEN

Reflections on the function of the skin in psychosocial space

Stephen Briggs

T he emotional responsiveness of parental figures to the containment needs of the infant is the starting point of the infant's development of an internal space and, thence, to a sense of his own coherence and identity. When parental responsiveness is impaired, the opportunities for experiencing internality and coherence are reduced. In this chapter I reflect generally on five observations of infants at potential (psychosocial) risk, drawing specifically upon one of these observations to suggest that Esther Bick's (1968, 1986) theory of psychic skin, and its function in early object relations, provides an extremely important conceptual tool for thinking about observations of infants in precarious or vulnerable social contexts.

The absence of containment—and often the presence of parental intrusiveness and projections into the infant—impacts powerfully on the infants. Elsewhere (Briggs, 1997a, 1997b), using an image of shape, I have described shifts in parental receptivity from Bion's (1962a) idea of reverie (concave), to parenting where the infantile communication is missed or blocked (flat), to that where the parental activity actively intrudes upon the infant (convex).

The impact of "flat" and "convex" parenting shapes on infants' struggles to develop inner resources in difficult and stressful circumstances is that particular patterns of relating emerge. My research suggests that in one of these patterns, infants seemed at times to develop a very muscular holding of the self. One infant, "Timothy", was almost gymnastic in the muscularity he displayed when mother moved away from him. Another infant, "Samantha", held her breath to the point of going rigid in mother's absence. For example, when she was 4 months 2 days: "Samantha looked blankly upwards, and shook a little. She put her fingers in her mouth and then held her breath, until she was quite rigid. She exhaled noisily again, her fingers held close to her mouth, going limp as she breathed out" (Briggs, 1997a, p. 161).

These examples illustrate the qualities that Bick (1968, 1986) described in thinking about the primary function of the skin. In the absence of containment the infant will try to hold himself together (Bick, 1986, p. 67 herein). A change of state—such as separating from the nipple or teat or taking off clothes when bathing—can induce a fear of a loss of psychic coherence, of falling apart, like being in "outer space without a spacesuit" (Bick, 1986, p. 66 herein). The anxieties of falling apart propel the infant to take action—a "frantic search for an object—a light, a voice, a smell, or other sensual object—which can hold the attention and thereby be experienced, momentarily at least, as holding the parts of the personality together" (Bick, 1968, p. 56 herein). The failure of the containing function of the mother could be observed through the "frantic search" for objects. Without someone or (by far second best) something performing the holding-together function, the infant has a "predominant terror . . . of falling to pieces or liquefying" (1986, p. 66 herein). In the face of this terror, Bick described gripping, grasping, and clinging contact and its meaning. Symington (1985) describes three ways in which the baby holds himself together: focusing on a sensory stimulus, engaging in constant bodily movement, and muscular tightening or clenching. Both Timothy and Samantha are examples of the attempts to hold the self through muscular activity, tightening, and clenching.

In these and indeed in all five infants in my study, the quality of holding together was observed distinctly and in quite extreme terms. Samantha's breath-holding experiences, observed on a number of occasions, had a particularly rigid quality. As well as these muscular, rigid attempts to hold the self together, there were also times when an infant would appear quite withdrawn, floppy, or blank. These infants seemed to have nothing to hold on to, in themselves or in other people, and there appeared to be a close link between a convex parental shape and a retreat to a withdrawn or blank state. Contact with others in these states was minimal and understated.

A very important question is how infants in disadvantageous social circumstances can develop inner resources. Thus, the meaning for the infants of their responses to the limited experiences of containment is crucial to their development. Yet in my study, it also emerged that infants developed, with some resilience, capacities to maintain or re-enter emotional connectedness in relationship with others. It seemed that there were links between the ways the infants found to hold themselves together, to survive (Symington, 1985), probably defensively, and the ways in which they continued to relate to others. Thus the possibility emerged of developing the theory of skin, to take into account the ways in which infants maintain development when containment is deficient.

Grip relations

If we take Bick's observation that the infant, in the absence of a containing object, seeks any object that will, even temporarily, afford some relief from the fear of internal disintegration, we can posit that the infant begins to seek a repertoire of objects, in ever more predictable ways, with different sensory modalities, in specific contexts. The quality, texture, and strength of the infant's contact with the mother, through the use of sensory modalities, will be very closely related to the kind of containment available. Bick suggested that the infant might use eyes, or voice, or the body, in a muscular way when a containing mother is not available. Bick's own observations were primarily concerned with the moments in which infants experienced a change of state or physical separateness.

If the focus is not only on the impact of separation, but also on moments in which contact is made—times of awakening, or reunion, for example—we can find examples in which the infant uses his initial "grip" on an object to create other "grips". For example, grips move from hand, to eye, to mouth. Dubinsky and Bazhenova (1997) provide examples of an "ascending" mode of contact. The infant gathers tone, integration, and unity in these moments of ascending grip relations. Having a grip on another is a precursor to the internalization of a reliable internal object (Williams, 1997b). On the other hand, when internal containment is fragile, infants may "exchange" one mode of contact for another, as the focus on one "grip" results in an incapacity to hold on to the other "grip" or contact through another sensory modality. Rhode (1997b) shows the effects of disjuncture between the eye and the mouth. Samantha, to whom I referred earlier, would fall down if she smiled. Smiling meant letting go of the rigid grip on herself, and her musculature that used to hold herself together; as a result, through smiling she exchanged a hold on herself for a contact with another.[1] Whether grip relations ascend or exchange at moments of contact in relatedness points to the quality of internalization of containment, the impact of excessive anxiety, and the restrictiveness of defences against anxiety. The example of Samantha's "exchange" of grip relatedness indicates a relationship between two emerging internal structures in the condition of limited containment. The first—holding the self together, rigidly—is a defensive attempt to survive; the second—a willingness to smile, and thus make contact with another—is a potentially costly experience with the consequence that she loses control of her musculature. The conundrum here is that without a firm or strong containing skin,

-----

[1] It is evident that, in this discussion, I am introducing quite a lot of recent thinking from child developmental studies, especially those studies that propose reciprocity (Brazelton, Koslowski, & Main, 1974), the readiness of the infant to communicate (Trevarthen 1998), and the capacities of infants to make use of perceptual apparatus in quite complex ways (Bower 1989). There are complicated distinctions between these studies and psychoanalytic approaches, and these distinctions are not always recognized when the wish to find congruence and convergence overlooks the essentially emotionally driven psychoanalytic formulations.

contact with others is costly and fraught. The greater the capacity for emotional contact with others, the less the risk to development; however, the greater the risk, the more is actually required of the infant to make and maintain contact.

The turn towards the emphasis on the quality of emotional contact with another marks a shift in psychoanalytic theorizing (e.g. Joseph, 1989) and reflects contemporary psychosocial dilemmas. A focus on grip relations in infancy makes it possible to follow the trends of the infant towards making and maintaining contact, and those trends away from contact. In infant observations, distinctions can be made between the kind of defensiveness that aims to sever contact (and possibly replace dependency on another with omnipotence), and that which aims, even in the stressful circumstances of limited containment, to maintain or restore emotional contact and dependent object relations.

From these observations I suggest that the term "grip relations" could be used inclusively to describe communications through any available sensory or perceptual modality, in order to express emotionality and relatedness. The meaning of these communications becomes of particular importance when infants, in considerable early difficulty in their social environment, become split between defensive withdrawal and attempts to maintain and sustain contact with others. Infants in difficult and stressful circumstances tend to "exchange" grip relatedness when relating to others, and the defensive aspects of grip relatedness become split from the channels that aim to make and maintain contact. For example, two infants in my study, both of whom were withdrawn rather than "muscular", developed a blank expression and made little eye contact. Contact with others was maintained by the use of the hand. Through the texture (loose, floppy, firm, or rigid) and the combinations or divisions of grip (ascending or exchanging modes of relatedness), the struggle between damaged and resilient parts of the self becomes visible, and poignant.

"Hashmat": an inter-cultural observation

I shall illustrate these processes through a discussion of one of the infants I observed, an infant in a precarious social situation. This is

Hashmat, the ninth son of Bengali parents. I have described the observation in greater detail elsewhere (Briggs, 1997a, 1997b); my discussion of it here is to illustrate how the application of the theory of skin and "grip relations" can be applied to development in vulnerable social circumstances, and, in this particular case, in a minority ethnic family. Understanding diversity is a priority for all engaged in contemporary therapeutic work with children and families, and this is a complex field where contexts of difference increase uncertainty of meaning. In this observational example, it is important to note how the quality of the family's vulnerability shifts between individual and cultural contexts, especially the encounter across cultures and the pressures of diaspora. For the minority ethnic family, there are imperatives to contend with negative experiences, and threats to a sense of belonging, and these produce ways of relating that provide a distinctive "social skin" (Healy, 1998). In Hashmat's case, I shall describe how limitations of parental containment and the qualities within a group culture "contained" both positive and destructive qualities. Thus, the characteristics of the family's "skin", as a function of survival, is a focus of the observations and provides a context for making sense of Hashmat's development.

The family

The context of difference was apparent from my first contact with this family. Hashmat's parents spoke very little English and they adhered strongly to a traditional way of life. The family size, the cultural difference between the family and the observer, and the fact that there was little common ground in terms of verbal communication created an unusual, ambiguous, and complex observational context.

The family home was a flat in a predominantly Bengali area of East London. "Javed", the father, speaking in Bengali through an interpreter (who was present for this initial visit only), said he was quite happy for me to observe. Indeed, he added, if I came later in the day I could observe all his children. They were aged 18, 15, 14, 13, 11, 8, 5, and 3 years. I said I would be pleased indeed to meet his children, but that I wished to concentrate on the new baby. Javed was quite portly, about 50, with a damaged eye. He did not work outside the home and throughout was a significant presence in observations. "Rani", the mother was darker skinned, with a warm smile, and she looked younger than her husband—under 40, I guessed. Both were traditionally dressed, and Rani's pregnancy showed very little. I wondered how I could obtain the mother's view of the observation and asked, through the interpreter and Javed, how they would feel about my observing, especially when mother was feeding the baby. Javed replied that his wife would not breast-feed. She had tried with the older children but did not have enough milk, and she would bottle-feed the new baby. He spoke to his wife, who nodded and smiled at me. The family appeared to welcome my interest in them. I was also sure that their motivation was more complex than this, and I wondered what I might come to represent for them. I also wondered how I might be able to under-stand, to try to avoid misunderstanding their communications.

Quality of containment

In this family, each member had a role and function in terms of parenting the baby. In order to think about the kind of containment experienced by Hashmat, I had to take into account the contribu-tion of the family members as a unit, as well as the quality of containment provided by Hashmat's mother. Two predominant and different family patterns were observed at different times dur-ing the observations.

First, and most prevalent, was a "group" culture, in which the primary notion was that any family member could look after the baby as well as anyone else. As the observer, I was initially invited to join this ideology, being asked to feed Hashmat, hold him, and be similarly involved with the other children. However, at times, rather than looking after the baby, the siblings would attack him, either physically or through inflicting an emotionally cruel situ-ation upon him. While father was noisily authoritarian, mother often delegated parental functions to the siblings. Both parents seemed unaware of the violence that erupted from time to time between the siblings and of the risk this incurred for the infant. Parental authority was absent when parents were physically ab-sent. At these times, the notion of a protecting parent, held in mind by the child, was also absent. The siblings joined together to gang up on the baby, and this had the impact of an intrusive, attacking, "convex" shape for the containing environment. At such times Hashmat was actually at risk, and on occasions I was forced to drop the more conventional observer role and actively intervene to physically protect either Hashmat or one of the younger children.

Second, by way of contrast, there were passages of time during which, with most of the older boys out of the house and both mother and father and two or at most three infants/young children in the home, the family resembled a nuclear family, where individual attention was possible. In contrast to the first pattern of relating, these passages seemed extremely peaceful and included interaction between parent and child, and play, but for large parts of the observation mother seemed quite passive and depressed, dealing with the very great burden of her situation by not thinking. If she did let herself think about the dependency needs of her children, she became easily overwhelmed and showed real helplessness. Her containing capacity was restricted because of these factors; in terms of her containing shape, she was mainly "flat".

As Hashmat's observer, I became engaged in quite complex exchanges with him, his parents and siblings, the extended family and friends, and the family's relationship to both British and Bangladeshi cultures. During the second year of observations, a cyclone in Bangladesh took many lives. Father left to visit Bangladesh, and the children were sick and anxious. The boys started to attack each other with sticks, without parental response. One of the older boys told me that "Bangladesh is slipping into the sea." The family's diasporic status and its meaning was thus poignantly described; the idea of Bangladesh falling into the sea conveyed a painful relationship with a culture through a metaphor that was imbued with infantile fears, of falling. This was particularly pertinent to the way I saw Hashmat develop, as I shall discuss.

Hashmat's early development

Hashmat's early development was remarkable because of his distinct defensiveness, retreat into a withdrawn state, which seemed closely connected with intrusiveness in the environment,

and a lack of individual space for him. His withdrawn state generated considerable anxiety about him in me as well as in the seminar
group where I discussed the observation. There were also some
communications to me from the mother and the older brothers that
he was not thriving, especially in that he would not take the bottle
and was often sick. There were some observations that showed that
he was making active efforts to survive and to maintain emotional
connectedness with others, albeit in a fragile and precarious way.

In the first observation, mother fed Hashmat, after father has
shown him to me. This is my first view of him; he is 9 days old:

> He has a shock of dark hair, pale fingers, and seemed delicate.
> Rani gave him the bottle, cradling the baby on her right arm,
> her large hand held out open-palmed. Hashmat took the bottle
> and sucked, closing his eyes. Rani looked at him and then at me,
> smiling a little self-consciously.

It is interesting to note from the beginning Hashmat's coordination
of mouth and eye, that his eyes closed when he found the bottle. He
has already learned from experience how to secure the bottle, but
it is not easy for him to locate both the bottle and mother's eye, or
mind. He seems to exchange one mode of contact for another.
Coordination of mouth and eye when feeding would not be an
expectation at this age, but the pattern continued, to become a
feature, whereby the idea that there is no eye—or emotional—
contact between them was jointly accepted. This way of feeding
was so regularly repeated that it held the quality of a sculpt. For
example, when Hashmat is 9 weeks:

> Rani looked up and smiled. She held him loosely, watching TV,
> her large hand open and then just touching his arm. His eyes
> were open and looking also in the direction of the TV. He
> sucked quietly.

The eye-seeking relationship and emotional contact when feeding
lie outside the mother–infant couple, in the "group", the family
nucleus. There are many objects of different qualities: the TV, in
this example, has a mindless quality. Father contributes a noisily
intrusive presence. "Shakil", the 3-year-old, is boisterous and mur-

derous, particularly when supported by the 5-year-old, "Chalaak". Mother wanted me to look after Hashmat, to employ me as she did the older siblings. When Hashmat was 7 weeks, she asked me, through one of the older boys, to feed him:

> I was in the room with Hashmat and three of the brothers. Mother entered the room carrying a bottle. She looked at me and spoke to "Miral", who is 14 years old. Miral, translating, said that Hashmat has been vomiting when feeding. I murmured sympathetically, and Miral went on to say that his mother would like me to try feeding him. He passed me the baby and mother passed a shawl. I held him on my lap and Miral went out returning with two tissues to catch the expected vomit.

While this presented me with a difficulty in role as observer, it also evoked father's comment that Rani had insufficient milk herself to feed the children. Overstretched with the demands of nine children, mother demonstrated, concretely, that she was not available at that time for Hashmat, either emotionally or physically:

> I was again holding Hashmat and I stood up as mother reappeared. I showed Hashmat to her and passed him to her. She held out her hands, palms up to prevent me giving her the baby, and gestured to Miral that he should take him.

Mother's unavailability was linked with the position, quite clearly derived from necessity, that the siblings should take an active role in holding, feeding, and responding to the baby. Frequently I was left alone in the room with Hashmat and his brothers. Play between the siblings Miral, Chalaak, and Shakil nearly resulted in Hashmat being injured.

> Hashmat began to cry. Wearily Miral went over to his cot and lifted him out, holding him in his arms, but continuing to play his wrestling game with Chalaak. Chalaak swung with his leg just missing Hashmat's face, and Shakil got Miral round the middle nearly toppling him and the baby. Hashmat stared wide-eyed away from them, his head on one side.

Hashmat was here an almost incidental presence in their aggressive games. The murderous intent was verbalized by Shakil when Hashmat was 8 weeks:

> Shakil started playing with a football. He said with menace, "No baby", and Hashmat lay with his eyes very slightly open as if peering or pretending to be asleep.

There was a constant theme of the lack of mediation of emotional experiences within the family or even acknowledgement of them. Hashmat's siblings were allowed in this way to give expression to their feelings of hostility towards the baby. Shakil graphically verbalized the idea that there should be "no baby".

Hashmat's defence against the intrusiveness and lack of containment was to withdraw. Repeated observations evidenced the experiences of assault on his bodily integrity, through noisy intrusion and the lack of emotional space for him in mother's mind. It became a very central question to think about how, in this context, he held himself together (Bick, 1968). He was not a muscular child, though I did notice on occasions he arched his back and stiffened, flapped his legs and arms, suggesting an unintegrated state. Often he seemed passive and withdrawn, his eyes glazed, and his movements minimalistically understated. Yet some small gestures showed he was surviving and was endeavouring to make or maintain relatedness. The most evident observations of his emotional survival focused on a complex relationship between his hand, himself, and other people.

We have already seen how his eye contact and the grip of his mouth on the bottle are kept separate, separating the relationship between feeding and relating (Rhode, 1997b). Now we can follow how he used his hand to make a grip on his world of relationships. First, when asleep at 11 weeks, his hand makes contact with the blanket:

> I watched Hashmat, and his hands touched one another so that the right one was resting on the left wrist. He was still for a time until he brought his right hand up and over his head; then he took it down and it caught the lip of the blanket. He shuffled this across his mouth. He twitched his head, eyes closed, from side to side and then cried.

This affords something of a precarious grip on himself, providing probably a phantasy or dream. He makes a grip with his hand on Shakil's finger and places his hands over his eyes as if to shield them. His hand grip is developing strongly, with variety. These quiet gestures, permitting some psychic survival, form prototypes of relationships which are seen throughout the observations.

In these early observations, I was struck by the contrast between the vulnerable Hashmat, whose development became so delayed, and the rumbustious pair of Shakil and Chalaak. Shakil has at times the attributes of a gangster; Chalaak is the epitome of toughness. Were they also withdrawn and fragile as babies, developing a tough "skin" to contend with this inner fragility, or is Hashmat different? Is Hashmat one boy too many in this family, or is there a family pattern whereby survival in a particular way—namely, of developing a tough, fighting skin—is part of the culture of development?

Development from 3 months to 12 months

Between 3 months and 12 months, Hashmat's behaviour was characterized by sudden spurts of development, which countered the feeling—and fact—that his development was markedly backward. He continued to seem remarkably unadventurous in his development and relationships with others. He was not sitting unaided until 8 months. Development occurred, as it were, from the outside. Parents put him in a bouncing-chair, and later a baby-walker, though he had shown no movement towards sitting up, raising his head, or trying to move about. But there were grounds for optimism. At 14 weeks, I saw him for the first time sitting in a baby-walker. This elevation was accompanied by a greater sense of curiosity. His hand grip was evident:

He looked alertly around the room and in my direction, his hair shaved and his very dark eyes looking out. His legs kicked a little and his arms moved also, his hands touching each other.

When I arrived for observations, he started to greet me with a smile and to seek me with his eyes. The relationship hinged on his hand grip, accompanied by his making sounds. For example at 4 months 2 weeks:

> Rani put Hashmat in the bouncing-chair, and went out, and he made high-pitched noises He seemed about to cry, and I leaned forwards and touched his foot. His hand reached down, so I put my finger in his hand and he held on to it tightly and pulled my hand towards him, and he made noises ranging between content, accompanied by a suggestion of a smile, to distress.

In this way he took some help in order to relate inner states of mind. Attempts at language and sharing a wide range of emotion followed, and a willingness to communicate continued. When he was 6 months 3 weeks:

> Hashmat sat and looked at me with a long look. His eyes focused on me steadily, with his face on the brink of tears. His hands moved on the table, and he had a small, hard plastic whistle which he held. He cast his eyes in the direction of the door where Rani had gone out. I smiled at him and felt there was something very delicate in his mood, so he could easily shift from smiling to crying. He made a little shrieking noise and I made a soothing one back. He put his finger in his mouth, and he poked with it behind his top gum, his mouth wide open. He took his finger out and held the toy which he dropped over the side. I retrieved it and he looked surprised to see it again, and he held it.

Here he seems to be communicating to me something about his teeth, to be saying "it hurts". My intervention is in tune with his preoccupation with absence. There followed a weekly ritual where he made lip-smacking gestures to me, which I imitated. His communication of pain is also seen when he was 9 months 2 weeks. Here the communication indicates the nature of the source of his distress:

> He is trying to crawl, but gets his leg caught. He cried a little and then gently banged his head on the floor some few times. Father then picked him up and after comforting him passed

him to me. He was hesitant and then touched my hand, grasping my finger, holding it quite tightly. He reached out to me and poked his finger into my mouth. He leaned against my chest and banged his head against it, lightly but with a feeling of wanting to make a space—concave—there.

Hashmat's interest in internal spaces, and his complaint that there is no space inside, is the first communication I have received that mother is pregnant. From the course of the observation so far, the state of pregnancy could be thought of as a metaphor for a mother who has no mental space for Hashmat's individual needs; now, at 10 months 17 days, there is evidence that he may be reacting to an actual pregnancy:

> Hashmat crawled under the table near Rani's feet, his head nearly touching the underside of the table top. There was no room for him to move unless he dropped down. He seemed to get stuck, and became motionless, frozen, unable to move. Rani's mother leaned down and gently pulled him out backwards, while Rani guided his head to stop it bumping the table.

This sequence has all the hallmarks of a role play of a forceps delivery, with Hashmat playing the baby and his grandmother the midwife.

My encounter with the family's experience of the birth of the new child, "Fashmat", a week before Hashmat's first birthday, was memorable. Father announced the birth in this way:

> Javed Ahmed came in and sat at the table and began to peel an onion with the curved knife. Then he said he may have to go to the hospital and added that his wife had a baby yesterday at 2.30 p.m.; another boy. He was looking pleased, a smile on his face as he spoke to me. Then he carried on peeling the onion.

Meanwhile, the children—Chalaak, Miral, and "Belal" (aged 11 years)—played a game of counting fruit:

> Belal said "apples, bananas, grapes, pears", and Miral added "apples, oranges, grapes, bananas, grapes", to which Belal re-

joined, with giggles "apples, oranges, grapes, pears, bananas, melon, grapes".

As the list grew longer and in random style, with repetition, one had the inescapable feeling that they were counting babies.

Hashmat's development continued in a somewhat covert manner. That this development had continued beneath a disguise of unadventurousness was made vividly apparent by the spurt in his development that coincided with mother's return from hospital. He was walking and speaking just before his first birthday:

> Javed Ahmed stood Hashmat on the floor and he walked a few steps towards us, and said "mama". Rani, with Fashmat on her lap, looked at him and smiled to me and repeated "mama".

Hashmat: development from 12 to 24 months

In the aftermath of the arrival of Fashmat and the adaptation of the family to another baby, Hashmat was faced with a choice. On the one hand, he could accept the family norm that babies are like fruit, and as common, and that the vulnerable, dependent attitudes of infancy should be abruptly and violently shed. On the other, he could maintain a relationship with mother, with all that this implied for experiencing individuality, uniqueness, and the capacity to communicate internal states of mind. The precariousness of this struggle is seen as Hashmat negotiated the passage between these two alternative ways of relating. Suddenly he was a toddler, not a baby. Developmental progress—taking his first steps and saying "mama"—gave him added capacity and separateness. It also confirmed his toddlerhood. He can now join the "gang" of brothers.

During this second year, he charted a course through three predominant states of mind. First, there was a boy in pain, who had the capacity to communicate his pain, demand a place with mother, and hold on to her. (There were occasions when I saw him standing by her, holding his hand on her knee—the hand continued to be important for him.) There was a developing curiosity. My presence was increasingly linked with this process. He became attached to some of the trappings of my role: my glasses, watch, and briefcase. The glasses seemed to symbolize my observing function. He wore them (in imitation of or identification with me) and explored their properties, touching them and looking through them. For example when he was 18 months 11 days:

> He climbed on the chair and sat next to me. He looked at my face, and then my glasses, and he gently leaned over and took them off. He passed them back to me. He took them off and passed them back, and I put them on. He did this again and put his face to the lens and sucked lightly.

The watch was clearly a symbol of my coming and going. He would come to me at the beginning of observations and ask to wear it. It appeared to help him work through the issue of separation and reunion. He was very curious about me, and his language began to develop. He seemed for a time to be bilingual, which amused Rani, who, when she was able to, watched his play benignly, and with interest.[2]

In contrast to this picture, Hashmat's second state of mind was aggressive and sadistic. He joined the "group", or gang, and his attacks focused on Fashmat (or a baby substitute) and the feeding bottle in equal measure. His shifts from one state of mind to the other could happen quite quickly, in the course of a single observation.

Hashmat's third quality of relatedness was characterized by a particular kind of withdrawal. He spent periods of time looking out of the window, in a rigid and "switched-off" mode. He became transfixed on these occasions, unaware of my presence even when I held him. This appeared to be a continuation of a withdrawn part of himself, which had been observed from very early in his life, whereby he became mindless in the face of external threats, depending on keeping a low profile in order to survive.

The following sequences from an observation when Hashmat was 15 months 1 week demonstrate both the shifts from one part of his self to another and the observer's role in providing a link between these states of mind.

---

[2] See Briggs (1997a, chapt. 9) for a discussion of the therapeutic role of the observer in these circumstances.

Mother showed Hashmat a tank on the living-room floor and moved it, playing. Hashmat pushed the tank and then stood up. Rani went out, and Hashmat looked at me and held his finger in his mouth with a pained expression. I imitated him and asked if it hurt. He smiled and moved his finger round his mouth. He moved across the room and picked up a toy, went to the doorway and picked up a belt and then turned round, looked at me, showed me the belt and went out of the room. I followed him and saw him throw some pegs on the floor. He came up to me, shaped as if to throw a tin he was holding and then passed it to me. I took it and passed it back.

So far, it is clear that Hashmat is closely connected in his mind with mother and me. He appears to think before he throws the tin and to use me to assist his thinking. When Fashmat appears, there is a change in Hashmat's state of mind:

The sound of Fashmat crying came into the room and Hashmat picked up the tin and went out of the room. He found mother and followed her into the living-room. Fashmat still cried. Hashmat climbed up on to the sofa and reached up to get his bottle, which was resting on the back of the sofa. He turned to me and held the bottle tightly between his teeth, pulling the teat. Rani looked at him and got up and fetched a pillow for him, seeming to understand what he wanted. She laid this on the sofa and sat down on the adjacent chair with Fashmat still crying, on her lap. Hashmat lay down on the sofa with the bottle and sucked it. He lifted his left leg up in the air and looked straight ahead and tensed his leg as he held it in the air. He twisted round so he lay on his side still sucking his bottle, which he held in his right hand, while his left hand covered his ear. Fashmat stopped crying but Hashmat still covered his ear. He twisted right round so he was lying on his tummy, his head on its side. He was now sucking more air than milk. He turned again and looked at Rani and passed her the bottle.

In this state of mind, he has to feed himself while mother feeds the new baby. He is muscular and tries with his body to hold himself together and with his hand to exclude the sounds of Fashmat crying. Then:

> Mother showed him a biro, and he climbed to his feet and slid off the sofa, landing on an empty lemonade bottle, crushing it. He exchanged the bottle for the pen and took it to one of the toys on the floor, bent over, and started to push the pen into a hole on the surface of the toy.

As the aggressor, Hashmat attacked the surface/skin in his play, and then his perspective reverses, so that instead of the aggressor he becomes the victim:

> I found him in the bedroom, kneeling on the bed and hanging out of the open window. I put him down on the floor and he protested, then he ran round the bed and came up to me with a smile and then sat next to me and I held him as he looked out of the window. He called out repeatedly "mama", pushing the window to and fro.

He was at risk at this point, when, in his mind, he was the subject of attacks on dependency, an infant needing mother rather than a ganging toddler. When he reverted to this position, he looked for a container, which was also holed.

Hashmat mimicked his older brothers. He imitated Shakil's tone of voice and the way the older brothers brushed their hair, and he got into Miral's shoes, literally:

> Hashmat had left the room, and now he came back in wearing big brother Miral's shoes. He grinned broadly and then seriously tried to concentrate on walking in them.

Hashmat is not trying on the shoes only for fun, he is aspiring to the status they represent—namely, a position in the family, and toughness. Herein lies an important aspect of the generation of a tough skin.

In the conflict between the siblings, humour and deadliness could follow upon one another. When the movement was from deadliness to humour, a sense of horseplay could be introduced

instead of grievous bodily harm. This was exemplified by
Hashmat's fight with Shakil when he was 18 months and 25 days:

> Hashmat followed Shakil, calling "oma" and "uhh". Gritting
> his teeth he hit Shakil on the back and arm. Shakil pretended to
> be dead and lay on the chair. Hashmat watched him and then
> hit him several times on the back, as if to stir him. Shakil got up
> with a big grin.

I found that as the observations continued and the two boys played
out their fights, I became less antagonized by the behaviour.
Moved by Shakil's humour, I found that I was thinking about the
difference between a playful, humorous interchange and its vi-
cious counterpart, a violent enactment. I wondered again how
toughness—the capacity to fight, to maintain a possession, or even
one's own body boundaries—was crucial to an infant developing
in these circumstances—*and* to the psychic survival of young Asian
boys living in contemporary British society.

Discussion

Hashmat's family occupy a very complex psychosocial space.
Alongside the capacity to make and maintain contact, the precariousness of Hashmat's early development led to a particular quality
of risk, and his resilience seems to be posited on a "tough" skin,
which has a sociocultural as well as an individual, psychological
meaning.

It is possible to see how Hashmat's early experiences are reflected in the characteristic states of mind he developed in his
second year, and the way these replicated earlier experiences. His
mimicry of his older brothers shows both an attack on the vulnerable, baby part of himself and his internalization of the group
culture of parenting, which began to place him in a particular
position with regard to others, having, that is, a distinctive social
skin. He seems to be actively administering to others that which he
had passively received earlier in his development. He becomes an
"insider", a member of the group—a brother—rather than an out-

sider, or baby. Alongside this, however, he maintained development within a context of dependency.

Both the limitations of parental containment and the qualities of the group culture had powerful impacts on his development. As I have said, in Hashmat's family the group "contained" both positive and destructive qualities. The attacks on babies, and the hostility towards dependent relationships, were particularly noticeable in the observations. However, located within the group was a system of development based defensively on sameness, and this functioned, often, on the brink, reflecting anxious diasporic ambiguities and uncertainties. The observation as a whole illustrates how careful attention paid to the meaning of grip relations can underpin understanding of the meaning of development within a specific psychosocial context, and one that is culturally different from that of the observer.

CHAPTER TWELVE

The skin in early object relations revisited

Judith Jackson & Eleanor Nowers

It was my [J.J.] privilege to be in Esther Bick's infant observation seminar for two years during the period when she was working on her ideas about the skin, and I remember how vivid and poetic were her descriptions of an infant's terrors of falling to bits, liquefying, when in an unheld, unintegrated, quivering state of unendurable being. I doubt that anybody else has ever given such resonance to what Bion (1962b) called "nameless dread". The seminar group was constantly enthralled by her detailed analysis of the many individual dramas unfolding, moved almost to tears by her unrivalled understanding of the poignancy of an infant's pain and helplessness, and shrivelled in shame when sharply confronted by our too-ready criticisms of a mother's shortcomings and difficulties. Her few papers are a pale reflection of her immensely gifted intuitions and creative thinking in pioneering the field of infant observation.

In this chapter, we would like to illustrate that drama and vividness through one such observation, beginning with some of the ideas contained in Bick's original, albeit very condensed, and complex 1968 paper regarding the primary function of the skin. In

this she describes the need of the unintegrated infant to be held .
together by the "skin" of the mother's containing functions.

> The thesis is that in its most primitive form the parts of the
> personality are felt to have no binding force among themselves
> and must therefore be held together in a way that is experi-
> enced by them passively, by the skin functioning as a bound-
> ary. But this internal function of containing the parts of the self
> is dependent initially on the introjection of an external object,
> experienced as capable of fulfilling this function. . . . Until the
> containing functions have been introjected, the concept of a
> space within the self cannot arise. Introjection . . . is therefore
> impaired. In its absence, the function of projective identifica-
> tion will necessarily continue unabated and all the confusions
> of identity attending it will be manifest. [1968, p. 56 herein]

Thus, there is an urgent need to search for a containing object—

> a light, a voice, a smell, or other sensual object—which can
> hold the attention and thereby be experienced, momentarily at
> least, as holding the parts of the personality together. The opti-
> mal object is the nipple in the mouth, together with the holding
> and talking and familiar smelling mother. [1968, p. 56 herein]

Bick, following Klein, emphasizes the importance of introjecting the mother's containing functions. Through this, the infant
becomes able to hold himself together in his own "skin", in the
absence of the external holding object, without spilling out and
falling to bits. There is an all-important double emphasis here: the
skin as a physical organ acting as a boundary between inside and
outside, self and object, literally holding the parts of the body
together, and the skin as a metaphor symbolizing the alpha-functioning and containing mind of the mother (Bion, 1962a) The ego,
as Freud (1923b) famously wrote, is firstly a bodily-ego.

In the face of any failure in this process, Bick describes how
the infant mobilizes ways of surviving or avoiding disintegration,
and she introduces the concept of a "second skin" to describe a defensive organization that provides a pseudo-independent modus
vivendi: a muscular or intellectual carapace, which offers self-containment but denies the need for the external object. This second-
skin conceals a fragile inner core and the faulty development of the

internalized "primal skin" of the mother, with all its physical and psychical properties.

How is the mother experienced in the inner world of a Bick baby? Can we hypothesize about the nature of the infant's primitive projective and introjective identifications with aspects of the mother? In the following pages, we attempt to describe an infant's use of his actual skin as a surface upon which can be inscribed, as it were, his early experiences, and we discuss how, through projective identification, his own manipulation of his skin might show a confusion with aspects of his mother which excite, frustrate, and envelop him. We are also interested in examining whether the development of a perverse, eroticized relationship to the skin serves as a kind of "second skin", resulting from the infant's attempts to defend against and master "a confusion of tongues" (Ferenczi, 1933) that he experiences as coming from his mother .

The infant observation of "Peter"

From the beginning of Peter's life, it seemed to the observer that he was held, and held together, in unconventional ways. As a newborn, he was laid uncovered on various surfaces, and when he was occasionally on his mother's lap, he was always at a distance from her body, not held closely by her arms, but intently scrutinized by her. His position was often precarious, and the observer feared he might fall, but the constant presence of either his mother's voice or her gaze apparently sufficed, and he seemed content. He made murmuring sounds in the short intervals in her endless flow of talk, as though dovetailing with it, and uttered loud, insistent noises if she temporarily left the room, in apparent protest at the absence of this holding, rocking voice. During the initial visits, the observer could perceive no desire for the breast on Peter's part and wondered whether his mother used the verbal and visual links between them to subdue any demand for the breast that he might make. The observer was repeatedly told *about* the breast-feeding— that it had just taken place, or was about to, or that it went on endlessly at night—but first observed a feed on her sixth visit. She, too, was to be satisfied by the mother's talk and spend the observations attending to her rather than the baby.

Observation at 6 weeks

The sixth time I visited, Mother fed Peter. She picked him up and, sitting him facing her on her lap, held him enthralled with her eyes and voice. He had an alert, wondering, even delighted expression when looking at mother and half-smiled in response to her. After some time Peter made urgent, repetitive noises as though he wanted something, and Mother commented that he wanted to be fed, but she didn't make any move to do so and continued talking to me. At last she laid him on his back across her knees. He immediately started making urgent noises, turning his head towards her and moving in an agitated way. Mother laughed and said he knew what this position meant. She seemed hesitant about starting to feed him but eventually lifted her jumper, whereupon Richard forcefully thrust his outstretched hand into her nipple. It caused Mother to flinch. She moved him closer so that he could latch on, and then he quietened, stopped moving, and fed steadily for some time. I could hear him gulping. Only his head and not his body was facing her. His arms were held in the air. Mother said that he would suddenly decide he had had enough, throw his head back, and go to sleep—she could tell if he had gone to sleep by his arm, which would slowly drop down as he dropped off. This is exactly what happened—his turned-away face creased up in an expression of satiety.

Peter's forceful striking of the breast caused the observer to wonder if the urgent fist were a substitute for the hungry mouth that could not yet reach the desired breast: a mouth/fist that had to plunge into the elusive nipple. The breast eventually gives up its milk, but the fact that it tantalizes and frustrates seems to provoke both the baby's initial violence and his later turning away from the breast as soon as he is sated. He throws back his head in a bodily gesture of rejection just as his instant falling asleep conveys a mental rejection.

During the next four weeks, his mother continued to delay his feeds, using a range of strategies that interposed herself, her voice, and her gaze between him and the breast. Aloud to the observer, she would give endless reasons why he shouldn't feed: he was full, he would be sick, he wasn't really hungry, and so on. Soon rather more active measures were required to quell the demands he was beginning to make. In the following observation, Peter was 8 weeks old and her voice and eyes had failed to stop his whimpers:

Observation at 8 weeks

After a few minutes delay she got up with a now very restless and whimpering Peter and suggested that they "do the aeroplanes" and then held him half at arm's length and circled him vigorously around her as she went out of the doorway. Peter went quiet and rigid, so she put him up on her shoulder as she went up the stairs.

The aeroplanes game in the doorway meant that his mother had to judge very precisely how to ensure his head did not hit the door-frame, and she responded to his apparent extreme alarm by cheerfully hoisting him into an exposed position. Once, after a series of delaying tactics, Peter suddenly began to scream with rage and frustration. Uncharacteristically flustered, M other crossly remarked that he could surely wait a little bit longer.

It soon became apparent that other needs of his were also being postponed, such as his need to sleep. During the day, Peter continued to nap in various places, uncovered on the armchair, on his changing mat, on their bed—allowed only a short time before being disturbed again. Sometimes he would lie balanced along her legs, and she would suddenly shift her position and wake him, as though to demonstrate his absolute dependence upon her. At night, she put him to bed before she was ready to sleep herself and, with equanimity, endured extended periods of his crying, only going upstairs when she believed he was asleep. Unable to let him feed or sleep as he wanted, her mothering strategies contradictory and unpredictable, over-impinging by day and abandoning by night, she became caught up in a perpetual oscillation between satisfying and frustrating his needs, which ensured that she remained the centre of her baby's universe, compelling him to adapt to her rather than the other way round. Nevertheless, passionate about her first baby and inseparable from him, she was proud of

what she thought was her natural ability to be a devoted mother,
and the observer realized that this mother was quite unaware of
what she was doing

The use of his skin as a location to register and express those
feelings that neither he nor his mother could mentalize began now
to come into play.

Observation at 10 weeks

Mother put him up on her shoulder to wind him. He went into
a little frenzy of rubbing his face against her shoulder, waving
his arms around as well, and kicking his legs. The strange thing
about it was how forcefully he scraped his face, such that when
we could see it again it had gone extremely red and sore.
Mother pointed out to me the tiny knots in his hair at the back
where he had rubbed his head on the sheet as he lay on his back
at night.

Peter had not fed to satiety. As he is winded, he seems to want
to rub into his mother as well as wanting to rub her out. There
seems to be a developing confusion between what is good and
what is bad, what he wants to take in and what he wants to expel,
what he desires and what he wants to attack—a confusion between self and object. Perhaps, as M other believed, the facial rash
causes the rubbing, yet observation implies that the rubbing
causes the rash.

During the observations between 10 and 18 weeks, Peter exhibited a growing irritability with his skin, while maintaining a contrasting alert and self-possessed facial expression. He rubbed his
feet together, or against the surface they lay on; he scratched at his
ears and the sides of his face where there were now sore patches.
The bald area on the back of his head had spread, and the rest of his
scalp was covered in red, pin-prick spots. His mother decided to
ration the breast and give him expressed milk by bottle instead,
and when he consistently rejected the bottle she responded by
offering solids. He rejected these efforts also, and feeding became a
dismal, dogged, and prolonged battle. The observer found it extremely painful to watch Peter's obvious wish to suck from the

breast frustrated, and it was soon it not only the alternatives that Peter pushed away, but also his mother.

Observation at 18 weeks

Mother lifted Peter into a sitting position and crouched right over him, cuddling him closely: his reaction was to fight her away with his hands. After this he put his hand to his ear and scratched irritably.

For a few minutes he angrily rubbed his head into her shoulder, butting her, but also as though his face was itching.

Observation at 5 months

He had been on Mother's lap and had attempted to feel for her breast through her jumper (*the observer thought he was hungry and wanted the breast*). She put him under his play-gym while she made us some tea. He concentrated on it for a few seconds and then seemed to have a little panic or frenzy, blindly hitting out, as though to hit away, the dangling toys. He calmed down and began to play with them again, and then again became agitated and hit out. This was repeated several times, as though he only just kept control of himself, or of something; as though he were on the edge of some panic, but just managing to recover himself and control the danger. He didn't appear to notice anything outside himself and his play-gym. He also scratched: dragging the toes of each foot down the top and inside of the opposite leg.

Peter seems to treat the toys as though they are like bits of the persecuting breast. Using his hands to reach out to them, he seems both to desire them and to need to fight them away, a distressed dilemma reflected in the way he uses his feet on his own body. During the next few observations, he continued to squirm away from his mother, refusing to look at her face or respond to her efforts to engage him, while engaging with his own body in the form of scratching. However, he sometimes reached for the withheld breast, or grabbed it through her jersey, and at these times his face would become suffused and red and he would go into little frenzies that conveyed both desire and hatred. The gaze that had linked him and his mother was now used by him to reject her: he would gaze through her as though she did not exist, or he would look away. The observer thought that both mother and baby were caught up in a tyrannical battle for control, each of them possessive, jealous, and painfully rejecting of the other. Trapped within this, it seemed that Peter had no emerging concept at all of his mother's separateness or absence, as all objects (like the toys above) were treated as though they were the breast.

These observations brought to mind Mrs Bick's ideas about the skin, as well as Bion's concept of an alpha-functioning mother. It seems that this infant has little sense of an external container able to process and give a meaning to his chaotic experience that he could introject. He is aroused and stimulated only to be frustrated; he is gratified when he least expects it, and he has no control over an unpredictable and wayward object. During this time his facial expression became characteristically impassive, solemn, and watchful, an outer poise appearing to reflect an inner state of readiness for whatever his mother might do next. His smiles were difficult to elicit and snatched back before he could dissolve into frank delight, and in between his little bouts of frenzy he became stiff and still. In marked contrast to this, his skin became increasingly volatile, visibly flushing and paling, and developing different rashes in different places. This culminated at the time of Peter's first separation from his mother at the age of 6 months, when his mother left him for a day with a friend while she made an essential family visit. The observer was shocked when she visited next day:

Observation at 6 months

He looked as though he had been badly burned. There were two large, raw, scarlet, weeping areas covering the top of each cheek, extending round his ears, and two similar areas, like crescents, on either side of his mouth. The rest of his face was covered in red blotches, and tiny raised red spots extended over his scalp. His general demeanour was a startling contrast: he was smiling broadly, interested and happy.

The shock that his appearance gives both his parents (and the observer) is the only evidence that Peter himself might have experienced any shock the previous day. His skin looks like "an envelope of rage" (Anzieu, 1989). We wonder if this extreme somatic reaction to separation from his mother further demonstrates that Peter has no sense of his own containing skin, since separation manifests itself in a mutilation that suggests that their mutual skin has been torn apart (Pines, 1980; cf. Di Ceglie & Di Ceglie, 1999). [1] His mother told the observer how good Peter was during his stay with her friend, and how proud she was of his ability to cope with being away from her, which again suggests that Peter has no conscious experience of separation from, or loss of, his mother, but that all is subsumed in his skin, which in his phantasy is also his mother's.

During the following months, Peter increasingly manipulated his own skin and flesh in a way that appeared to demonstrate a desperate effort to master the experiences he had to survive. He stopped putting on weight, which eventually led to an alarmed intervention by the health visitor. Mother was outraged that her mothering abilities were called into question, and she indignantly interpreted the situation as demonstrating how sensible her child was only to eat as much as he wanted, rather than greedily cramming himself full like other babies. Observation showed a very different story. On innumerable occasions Mother would interrupt a feed or a meal by coming between Peter and his food: she would remove the bottle or spoon and rub noses instead, "empathically" decide he was feeling full, discover the teat was blocked and forget to unblock it, or even eat his solids herself. In all cases, however, she could then present herself as the object her son really wanted. As this situation continued, Peter showed fewer and fewer signs of

---

[1] Britton (1999) comments: "Certainly, it is my experience of some borderline patients that there are passages in analysis when it seems as though analyst and patient only had one skin between two with the risk that someone might be skinned alive" (p. 24).

hunger, thus appearing to justify his mother's version of events. His collusive indifference to being starved was belied, however, by his increasingly violent attacks on his skin, suggesting evidence of early splitting mechanisms.

Observation at 7 months

He clawed at his abdomen, pulling up the skin into folds in his hands and squeezing it before letting go and then doing it again. He wriggled and kicked, looking at his mother and smiling, and continued to rake his tummy with his hands as though he would wrench off bits of flesh.

Observation at 8 months

Peter used both hands to grab his genitals, squeezing them and then wrenching upwards with his fingers curved into his testicles. It looked very painful, but his face remained impassive. He grabbed the fat above the genitals and twisted it so that the area went bright red, with raised patchy weals extending up his abdomen. He was too intent on this to play with the soft toy that the observer offered him because she couldn't bear what he was doing.

Peter rarely rubbed or scratched at his skin alone, but tore, raked, yanked, twisted, clawed, squeezed, and wrenched both his skin and the flesh below it. His hands performed these actions on himself while his smiling or expressionless, wide-eyed face made a bizarre contrast. An onlooker would imagine that the sensations the baby must have produced on himself would be painful, even unendurable at times, but Peter's demeanour conveyed self-absorption and even narcissistic pleasure, and it was clear that he would deliberately choose to move from a savaged area of skin to an unmarked one. In other words, it seemed that as an area of skin became less sensitive to his attacks he tried to extend the sensation as much as possible, as though to provide himself with this perverse sensation as a form of containment. Sometimes it seemed that he did this most urgently in situations where he might be expected to fear a falling apart—for instance, when naked after a bath and left alone in his room while his mother let out the bathwater.

By digging into his flesh, Peter must now have been arousing sensations far deeper than the skin, and so we also wonder if he was creating a bodily experience of being both the "container" of the body and also "the contained", an all-body confusion with his mother. Segal, in her paper "Notes on Symbol Formation" (1957), writes that "The early symbols . . . are not felt by the ego to be symbols or substitutes, but to be the original object itself" (p. 164). It seems possible that Peter's own skin and flesh is a symbolic equation with his mother's. This implies that in terms of his mental development, Peter was unable to progress to the stage in which true symbolization occurs; in other words, there was a difficulty in even beginning to negotiate the depressive position, with its attendant fear of loss and guilt, and eventual recognition of the mother as a separate person with her own body and mind.

The operation of a violent projective identification with his mother also may be seen in the way his grabbing of his own body mimics in somatic terms his experience of his mother's behaviour towards him. Through projective identification he inhabits her, as it were. In a further twist, just as her variably tantalizing, depriving, and sadistic behaviour occurs concurrent with her devotion, so does Peter spare his real object even as he attacks it in his own body through its use as a symbolic equation. Each inflicts cruelty upon the other, and yet both preserve their "skin-deep" mutual equanimity and contentment.

The function of the skin

The use that this baby might be making of his skin is already very complex. First, it acts as a location to express his responses to his *external* environment: it flushes and pales, or develops spots and rashes.

Second, it has appeared to act as a screen upon which *inner* psychic response can be projected—for instance, the dramatic skin reaction when he was separated from his mother. As a preverbal and apparently consciously contented baby, it is his skin only that seems to manifest the inner psychic turmoil that emerges in the shocking appearance of his skin, which seems to suggest early massive splitting, where the psyche-soma reveals two quite different states of mind.

Third, we have described the manipulation of his skin to provide an auto-erotic sensation of containment, and maybe also of his flesh, to provide a sensation of that which is contained.

Fourth, through projective identification it seems he uses his body as a symbolic equation. Thus he becomes his goading, unpredictable mother in relation to his own body and, in addition, is able to inflict his phantasied desire and rage on that same desired but frustrating mother. We have wondered what this might tell us about his stage of psychic development.

A perverse relationship

All the complexities that have so far been perceived in this infant observation form a dramatic backdrop to the development of a perverse relationship with the precariously containing mother whom, through projective identification, he now so vividly echoes. The stage is set for what seems to be this infant's sadistic masturbatory engagement with himself, mirroring his experience of his mother's perverse relationship with him. She continued to dote on the son she happily described as so contented and laid-back, and she remained oblivious both to his starvation and his emotional pain. She viewed his reddened and injured skin as eczema and took great pains to treat it with soothing creams, which she massaged into him morning and night. Peter appeared to dislike this gentle touch, and he wriggled and pushed her hands away so as to resume his rough manipulation (frequently masturbation) of himself instead. His apparent preference for painful rather than gentle treatment reflected his mother's preference for "doing aeroplanes", or swooping and bouncing her baby rather than cuddling or rocking him. Furthermore, his mother responded to his attacks on himself, particularly when it was on his genitals, with her own reciprocal excitement, and there were frequent skin-to-skin encounters between them, particularly around bathtime when Peter was naked, during which each performed on the other the clawing, poking, twisting (and biting) actions, as though as an expression of their mutual passion and devotion. At such times she occasionally cupped and shook his genitals, or got him to sit on her hand so that she could mock-reprove him, and she used coarse sexual endearments to address him. These encounters usually ensured that the appropriate need of the baby was sidelined:

Observation at 8 months

He drank from the bottle, stretching out his hands and feeling for his mother's face, trying to get his fingers into her mouth, pulling at her lips. She seemed to enjoy this, mock-complaining, making noises, dropping her face to kiss or nuzzle him. The play started gently enough on Peter's part, but soon became more active, at times frenzied. He stopped sucking, and they played with each other, the bottle pushed out of the way,   his mother butting into his body and neck, he aiming for her face with hands. Then there seemed a similarity between what his hands were doing to his mother and what he does to his own body when he is naked: he wanted to twist, stretch, compress, and tear.

Here, once again, the food gets mislaid. Peter's experience of desire (both for food and to explore gently his mother's body), need, frustration, and deprivation becomes subsumed into an exciting, rough, sensual experience that joins the two of them together and becomes its own gratification,[2] perverse because it is a substitute for his real needs. What his hands perform on his own skin and on that of his mother condenses his complex mental state with a substituted gratification, while sustaining a contact with a mother who loves, but misunderstands, him.

Peter's muscular efforts in relation to himself, or to his mother, visibly and intensely engaged his entire body, and this was in marked contrast to his otherwise retarded motor development. In

---

[2] This could be seen as a precursor to the development of perverse states of mind as seen in adult patients who use sexualization as a defence against real relating, which implies separateness from the object (cf. Freud, 1910i; Joseph, 1994)

the months when he might be expected to make efforts to roll, crawl, or stand up supported by his mother's hands, he just about managed to stay sitting, and otherwise was passive and inert. The observer wondered if this reflected an instinctive strategy to conserve energy at a time when he was underfed and failing to thrive, and she also thought that it was an extension of the alarmed and watchful attitude that began very early on: to meet his mother on her own ground required his absolute attention. His denial of the dependence and deprivation that was his actual predicament seemed particularly evident during mealtimes, when he showed an alarming indifference to the presence of food but could throw himself into an intensely energetic encounter with his mother.

The significance of a father's role

Up to the age of 9 months, Peter and his mother seemed mesmerized within an exclusive relationship. Peter's father usually worked long hours, but he was suddenly unemployed for several weeks. His constant presence in the house during this time appeared to rupture the skin within which his wife and son were trapped, and the observer witnessed a dramatic transformation in Peter.

Observation at 10 months

Peter looked past me at his father, smiled broadly, and crawled rapidly to him, brushing past my legs without a glance at me. His father greeted him affectionately and picked him up. Peter settled himself in his father's arms, looking pleased, and then looked at me. His father didn't actually play with Peter, but at ease with each other, they just were . . .

Peter and his mother seemed rescued by the active involvement of his father, and both exhibited relief and freedom. The invisible bonds that had prevented Peter's motor development fell away, and he began crawling and exploring his environment with purpose and pleasure; he began experimenting with sounds, babbling to himself as he played, and, most reassuring of all, he put on weight. His mother happily described it as "the onset of a new era", as though at some level of her mind she realized something malignant had been thwarted, and she was glad to accept her husband's help in looking after Peter. The observer thought it significant that mother chose this time to think about becoming pregnant again.

Peter's discovery of his father seems important because the father is a safe, reliable, and loving presence that provides an essential alternative to his mother. Peter could now become aware of separation and difference from his mother and was freed to move and explore. The sense of being held together by a whole skin seemed to be evoked now by the act of very fast crawling, or by being in enclosed spaces such as behind the sofa, the curtains, or a ladder propped against the wall. In such places, as in his father's arms, he would settle himself and look around with a pleased smile, sometimes then pushing hard to produce a usually constipated stool. He became more solid and more comfortable in his own body, and instead of using his own skin as the major means of expressing his perverse entrapment and control over his internal and external relationship with Mother, he made use of more appropriate spatial enclosures, allowing for symbolic play. The vicissitudes of the depressive position were no longer held at bay.

The observer noticed that he would often make for his father (and in father's absence, his office!), but that he preferred to keep a distance between himself and his mother:

Observation at 11 months

He slithered off her lap, pushing the bottle away, head averted. She let him go and he crawled rapidly to the other side of the room. She put him on her lap and offered the bottle again, and at first he accepted it. Only a few minutes later he rejected it as firmly as before and raced off across the room again.

However, mother and son sustained their vocal contact at a distance, this "sonorous envelope" (Lecourt, 1990) remaining a constant in their subsequent relationship:

Observation at 12 months

There was a curious conversation between them, as Peter looked at his toys. His mother was saying any old thing for a sentence, dead-pan, and Peter answered her with a variety of cadences that tended to mimic hers. On her part it was all rather patronising, as though she might throw me a wink about it all. She remained at the other side of the room from him, yet her voice never left him alone.

At times it seemed to the observer that Peter used the "conversation" between them to lull them both into a sense of mutual need and gratification while he got on with the business of growing up by making use of what she could and did provide for him. Now busy and verbal, Peter's use of his skin largely ceased, and although he still scratched sometimes while eating and drinking, or at bathtimes, his skin was almost entirely clear by the time he was 1 year old.

Peter at the age of 10 years

In her original paper, Bick writes that " the faulty skin-formation" produces a general fragility in later integration and organization. Any infant observation, including the one from which we have drawn our material for this chapter, inevitably arouses curiosity and concern about the future development of the observed infant. What will characterize the child, the adolescent, and the adult that the baby will grow up to be? As a 10-year-old, Peter was thin, quiet, watchful, and sensitive. Although he was not particularly outgoing, he was very good at athletics. He hero-worshipped his kind but firm father whom he tended to obey; he was wary, sometimes defiant, in his mother's volatile and ever-verbal presence. He was protective towards his boisterous younger siblings. Liable to be teased at school, he could wrap himself up in an imaginative world and enact it through play. He spoke in a halting but quietly determined way. He was slow in learning to read and write and was diagnosed as suffering from a mild form of dyslexia. This raises the question of whether a repressed, unconscious failure in the internalization of a containing maternal "skin" might have an effect upon the ability to perceive accurately the relationships between letters, words, and sentences—the physical "skin", as it were, of meaning. Throughout his childhood he showed a tendency to suffer from a recurrent unexplained malaise characterized by aches and pains and fatigue, which might suggest that an early use of the body to express and contain psychic pain may predispose to psychosomatic complaints throughout life (McDougall, 1985). An intriguing aspect of his later development, therefore, is his continuing vulnerability, as shown through his shyness, the dyslexia, his propensity to being teased, and his somatic complaints. What does this say about the maintenance of his "second-skin" formation? Is there a location for the cruelty experienced by him and enacted by him upon his own body? As an older child, he seems thin-skinned and not thickskinned; a "fragile inner core" is evident and not concealed. Perhaps the cruelty he experienced, which he then enacted upon his own body, is in a hidden location, or "holed up in the body" (Coltart, 1986), waiting to emerge at an even later stage in his development. Alternatively, can we see an over-tender alliance with his objects instead? [3]

Conclusion

In this chapter, we have taken as our starting point Bick's thesis concerning the overriding importance of the function of the skin. We have used the observation of one infant–mother couple to describe the various ways in which one infant has used his skin to express, contain, and control psychic pain and his unconscious experience of the failure of his mother's "primal skin function". Despite the perversity evident in what we have described, we think it important that through his use of his skin he revealed a vital and creative part of himself, searching for a way to survive— an engagement with life clearly evident ten years later.

---

[3] "The special interest of psycho-somatic symptoms . . . is that the rough beast whose hour is not yet come is holed up in the body. . . . Mostly he seems inaccessible, and we perceive that part of the mind has lodged in a psychotic island in the body" (Coltart, 1986, p. 198).

We have also highlighted and demonstrated the importance of following the detail of repeated patterns of interaction which fill out a picture over time, showing how such patterns have the potential to become entrenched in the psyche-soma from the moment of birth. Bick (1964) emphasizes this in her paper on the importance of infant observation in psychoanalytic training:

> The point that I am stressing here is the importance of consecutive observation of the individual couple. The experience of the seminar is that one may see an apparent pattern emerging in one observation, but one can only accept it as significant if it is repeated in the same, or a similar, situation in many subsequent observations. Paying attention to such observable details over a long period gives the student the opportunity to see not only patterns but also changes in the patterns. He can see changes in the couple's mutual adaptation and the impressive capacity for growth and development in their relationship, i.e. the flexibility and capacity for using each other and developing which goes on in a satisfactory mother–baby relationship.   [p. 47 herein]

CHAPTER THIRTEEN

Whom does the skin belong to? Trauma, communication, and sense of self

Maria Rhode

In "The Experience of the Skin in Early Object Relations", Esther Bick stressed the "catastrophic anxieties in the unintegrated state as compared with the more limited and specific persecutory and depressive ones" (1968, p. 56 herein). Overcoming the total helplessness of unintegration and moving on to achieving the necessary split between good and bad, she wrote, depended on the "earlier process of containment of self and object by their respective 'skins'." Failing such containment, experiences of falling forever and of spilling out—of feeling lost in "outer space without a spacesuit", as she put it in her second paper on the experience of the skin (Bick, 1986)—might be defended against by "second-skin" coping devices in which the baby holds himself together by the "inappropriate use of certain mental functions" of his own. Bick's clinical examples include people who make use of their athletic or verbal capacities in this way. One of the patients she described alternated between a fragile "sack of apples" state in which he was constantly expecting catastrophe, and a "hippopotamus" state in which he was "aggressive, tyrannical, scathing, and relentless in following his own way". "The 'hippopotamus' skin," she wrote, was "... a reflection of the object's skin inside which he existed, while the thin-skinned, easily bruised, apples inside the sack represented that state of parts of the self which were inside this insensitive object" (1968, pp. 58–59 herein).

My aim in this chapter is to explore some of the experiences that may be associated with realizing that the self and object do indeed have their respective skins—that the mother's skin marks the boundary of her own separate body. This boundary—the fact of physical separateness from the mother (Tustin, 1972)—may be seen by the child as being the cause of any pain he suffers. Sometimes mother and baby can seem to be competing for the skin as for something essential that protects them and makes them feel complete. When this is so, problems can arise for the therapist who attempts to interpret catastrophic anxieties: the child can misunderstand her capacity to think about them and to put them into words, as though she were flaunting her possession of the very thing he lacks and feels to be essential. In the case of a traumatized little girl whose material I shall discuss, such a misunderstanding made for considerable technical difficulties.

First of all, I wish to review some theoretical links between Bick's conceptualization of catastrophic anxieties and the work of other authors. In France, Anzieu's writings on the skin-ego (Anzieu, 1985) have led to a rich exploration by many workers of various forms of primitive containment—of the way in which "psychic envelopes" come into being (Anzieu, 1985, 1987; Kaës & Anzieu, 1993). In Britain, Bick's formulations within the Kleinian tradition clearly touch on some of the same areas as do Winnicott's explorations of the catastrophic anxieties (Winnicott, 1949) which can stem from deficiencies in maternal holding. One main difference is that Bick stresses the mother's toleration and containment of infantile anxieties, while Winnicott (1951) emphasizes that, in the very early stages, the mother should provide an environment that does not confront the infant with the fact of his separateness.

The other fundamental link is with Bion's theory of containment and maternal reverie (Bion, 1962a). As is well known, he proposed that the catastrophic terrors suffered by parts of the infant's personality could become meaningful and bearable through being projected into the mother, whose personality had to be strong enough to tolerate and contain them. That part of the infant's personality which he had been unable to own could then be integrated once it had been "detoxified" during its sojourn in the mother's psyche. It will be evident that Bick's formulations concern the physical counterpart of the psychic processes described by Bion. She too emphasizes the central importance of the mother's ability to tolerate and process aspects of the infant's personality: this is what allows the infant to feel that these parts are held together by a skin that is both physical and psychic. Geneviève Haag (1991, 2000) has extended this line of thought in her description of what she calls the " *boucle du retour* ", in which the baby experiences his emotional communications as gaining access to the mother through her eyes and as travelling through her head until they come up against the back of her skull. The latter is a vital step in the process: in the absence of this boundary the communication could be imagined as travelling on indefinitely and getting lost in space, as with a mother who does not respond. With a responsive mother, however, the infant's message encounters the "foundation" of the back of her head and passes back out to the infant through her eyes, having been transformed by its sojourn in the mother's head.

Such a statement of the physical concomitants of Bion's concept of containment points up the way in which the baby's sense of his own coherent boundaries is grounded in the experience of the mother's skin boundary. When all goes well—when emotional communication by means of eye contact is unimpeded—the mother's boundedness becomes the foundation of the baby's own sense of a bounded self contained by a mental and physical skin. When things go wrong, this may be experienced as the mother's failure to receive the baby's communication; as a failure to meet it, so that it goes off into space; as a failure to provide the needed emotional transformation; or as a failure in the way the communication is returned to the baby (in the clinical situation, this includes the timing of an interpretation). All these failures may be construed or misconstrued in various ways by the infant or patient and have been described by many authors, including Bion (1962a), Joseph (1975), Alvarez (1992), and Britton (1998c). These failures in emotional interaction will all have correlates in terms of how the child experiences his own skin in relation to the skin boundary of the mother—whether in terms of maternal impermeability, damage to the maternal boundary, failure to constitute the child's skin because of inadequate containment, or intrusion by an aspect of the maternal boundary.

This leads me on to the masculine aspect of the containing function. Recent papers by Didier Houzel (2001a, 2001b) beautifully illustrate the essential role of what he calls the bisexuality of the containing object in permitting a child with autism to integrate his own masculine and feminine elements. The central position of the father in presiding over the child's entry into what French psychoanalysts call the symbolic order has been approached from a somewhat different perspective by writers in the Kleinian tradition. Meltzer (1967), for instance, talks about the breast as having a feminine receptive component combined with a masculine element, the nipple, which he suggests is experienced as the guardian and protector of the breast, the guarantor of its separateness and integrity. Sydney Klein (1980) has differentiated the baby's earliest experience of the father element as supportive from a later experience of an intrusive father, while Resnik (1995, pp.102, 106) emphasizes the importance of the *"père pontifex"*, the father who functions as a solid bridge, which protects the child from being engulfed by the mother. Britton (1989) has documented the centrality of the oedipal triangle, experienced on an archaic level as well as on the level of whole, separate people, for the constitution of mental health and the capacity for thought. These conceptualizations may readily be linked with Bion's delineation of the various components of maternal reverie: "feminine" receptivity towards distressed parts of the infant; the digestion and transformation of the experience that the infant needed to evacuate; and the active, "masculine" function of returning to the infant of the transformed part of its personality. "Masculine" or "feminine" are, of course, here a matter of psychological functions, not of the gender of the person performing them. In terms of the physical correlates of Geneviève Haag's *boucle du retour*, one could say that the mother's eyes perform first a feminine function in receiving the infant's communication, and then a masculine function in returning it once it has been transformed.

Although these ideas can appear complicated, small children talk about them quite naturally. For example, baby "Rachel" at the age of 20 months was observing a row of milk bottles with red foil caps. Pointing to each cap in turn, she said, "Daddy . . . daddy . . .

daddy." Here is the paternal aspect of the skin function that guards the integrity of the bottle, prevents the milk from spilling, and protects the child from being flooded or engulfed. On the other hand, the notion of the mother's skin as the prototype of all obstacles is illustrated in the words of another little girl, who said to her mother, "I hate your skin because it stops me getting right inside you." "Getting inside" may feel particularly urgent if the mother is emotionally preoccupied: children with autism, in particular, often seem to misunderstand their caretaker's mental preoccupation to mean that she is physically occupied by someone else (Rhode, 2000; Wittenberg, 1975). Unwelcome emotional experiences that intrude into the child can be mistakenly attributed to the paternal element—one boy with autism had a good relationship with men on a one-to-one basis, but if he and I together met up with a man coming towards us, he always reacted by covering his ears as though to protect himself from a loud noise (Rhode, 1997a). Observations of this kind make it understandable that a child who is being projected into (Williams' omega function: Williams, 1997a) can develop a concept of a bad father even when no father is present in external reality.

An observation of baby Rachel—the little girl with the milk-bottle tops—at the age of 3 months may serve to illustrate this experience of being intruded into, followed by what looked like an attack on the mother's skin boundary, which in turn led to problems with the baby's own skin.

> Baby Rachel had had to spend a night or two in intensive care immediately after birth and had been subjected to some intrusive and painful medical procedures. Although she and her mother left hospital at the normal time, she cried a great deal, was difficult to settle, and tended to cling to the breast for reassurance. Her mother developed cracked nipples and was advised to take the baby off the breast to allow them to heal. Her milk supply decreased as a consequence, so that Rachel required supplements; since she persisted in refusing a bottle, her breast-feeds were supplemented with milk from a spoon, which took a long time and meant that she had to be very patient. In the observation I wish to refer to, Rachel rested for a moment after she had finished drinking from the spoon, then

gripped the skin on the back of her mother's hand and twisted it hard. The observer thought that if Rachel had been bigger, she would have left a mark. When the observer returned for the next observation a week later, Rachel had developed eczema.

Here, then, is a baby who was not yet developmentally ready for the move to the spoon, which involves tolerating the discontinuity between the mouth and the source of food. Following O'Shaughnessy's (1964) conceptualization of Bion's model as "good breast absent equals bad breast present", Rachel appears to experience the spoon as the incarnation of the absent nipple, and we could speculate that the discontinuity that the spoon imposes on her might mean that it becomes for her something intrusive that pokes into her mouth. This may well link with the intrusive medical procedures that she suffered in the first hours of her life, and which, together with her parents' anxiety, may have been a factor in her clinging to the breast as though it were a dummy. This single observation does not permit us to differentiate between the likelihood that Rachel experienced the unwelcome spoon as an extension of the skin barrier on her mother's hand which she then attacked, and the alternative possibility that Rachel felt responsible for her mother's cracked nipples and was testing this out on her skin. In either case, it seems plausible that Rachel's eczema was a sign of her identification with her mother's twisted skin, not just an expression of her experience of inadequate containment.

The next vignette I wish to discuss concerns "Anthony", an 11-year-old boy with autism, who had just missed a treatment session in order to go to a musical he had long wanted to see. When his mother discussed with him that this would mean missing a session, he had said to her that Mrs Rhode was going to be ill on that day.

On the way to the therapy-room, Anthony tried to continue up the clinic stairs instead of stopping at the second floor where the therapy-room was located. This had happened before, and we had talked about it in terms of his wish to grow up and the feeling that I was holding him back by keeping him on the second floor. When I linked this to his having a good time away from me, and his difficulty in thinking that I would not mind, he regressed to miming the agonized birth of a baby whose head seemed to be bitten off while passing through the crack between the cushions on his chair. This, too, was a familiar constellation. I said to him that I thought he went back to being a baby in danger of death when he could not believe that growing up and doing things he liked would not make me ill. Did he really think, I asked, that having a good time would make me ill and upset me? Quite exceptionally for him, he answered directly—"No"—then went to lie on the sofa, pulling a chair on wheels against it to make sure he did not fall off the edge. He then pulled the sofa-covering off and wrapped himself in it. I said perhaps he could not believe he could feel protected without pulling the cover off the sofa, as though there could be a skin either for him or for me, but not for both. (I should add that there was a blanket available, so untucking the sofa covering was not the easiest option.) Much to my delight, Anthony responded by pushing the chair on wheels over to me. For the first time in his treatment, a game developed in which we pushed the chair back and forth between us, and when I suggested a game of catch with his ball he was able to join in this for some time. Quite suddenly, he gripped hold of the ball and of a roll of sellotape which he held up against his face while staring at the ceiling: he was no longer able to play and was unavailable when I attempted to explore this.

Anthony's loss of the ability to enjoy the to-and-fro of the ball between us, his need to maintain his grip on it, seems linked to a sudden fear of distant objects and of three-dimensional space. Bick (1968, 1986), Tustin (1972, 1981a, 1981b) and others after them have described the degree of terror—primarily the terror of falling—with which three-dimensional space can be associated. Indeed, the roll of sellotape that Anthony clutches to his face may serve as a reassurance against the perspective of the distant ceiling. On a more developmentally evolved level, it seems possible that he was hallucinating onto the ceiling something that interfered with his having a good link with me. What I chiefly wish to emphasize, however, is the way he seemed to feel that he and I were in rivalry for a position of happiness, security, and competence, much as Tustin's patient David felt that he built himself up by concretely cutting bits off his father (Tustin, 1972). In Anthony's case, it was the skin-like sofa cover that seemed to be the essential piece of equipment, and his ability to join in the to-and-fro of a game of catch, to share the ball with me to our mutual benefit, followed immediately on the interpretation of his fear that if he had a skin it must mean tearing mine off me.

Against the background of these two vignettes, I wish to discuss some skin-related aspects of the therapy of a little girl between the ages of 3½ years and 5 years.

"Clara"

Clara's parents were at their wits' end because of her sleeping difficulties. She woke several times every night in a state of terror, did not recognize her parents, and could not be comforted. During the day she was extremely clingy and controlling in a way that came over as very aggressive. Work with a colleague had strengthened the parents in setting limits, and when I saw them the mother had just become pregnant.

The history the parents told me was a painful one. They were a united couple who coped with father's frequent absences on business by a mixture of courage, denial, and immersion in their respective careers. There had been a miscarriage before Clara, so they were overjoyed when she was born, though understandably more anxious than they might have been in other circumstances. Mother's description of a happy time of closeness when Clara was a baby occasionally suggested a blissful union in which father's absences hardly impinged. However, his work meant that the family had to move to London. They described their new flat as horrible, in stark contrast to the flat they had left behind, and it seemed to epitomize all their feelings of being uprooted. Then mother suffered another miscarriage, and Clara contracted a life-threatening illness. She had to be hospitalized, and though she made a full physical recovery, her parents had not recovered emotionally from the fact that she could have died.

Clara was tiny and delicate, pale and fair-haired with big, blue-grey eyes. At 3½ years, she was fine-boned and slim-waisted, a miniature version of her mother, with no remaining baby roundness. Her clothes, whether party dresses or jeans, were exquisite and fashionable. In the assessment sessions, she organized her parents to execute her ideas, as though they were children being guided by a strict but kindly teacher. They complied without a murmur, and she was clearly not pleased with me when she asked what I wanted to play and I said that we were there to do what she chose. Owning any kind of desire seemed quite impossible. She set her parents to work softening the plasticine, then instructed her mother to "make a little fellow", and she made sure that the little fellow contained some of mummy's plasticine in combination with some of daddy's. She showed us seriously that the little creature was complete—he had eyes, nose, mouth, ears, all his fingers and toes, as well as a willy. This was obviously a very serious matter for her, and her manner during this part of the session was in complete contrast to her prevailing manner of perfect poise verging on irritatingly controlling bossiness. Alongside this she showed us primitive anxieties about falling and spilling out: toys got dropped over the edge of the table; the beaker of juice she had brought with her came apart and spilled and she urgently asked for the lavatory. In later assessment sessions, I had to take the part of a naughty child who had committed a serious fault, though without being told what it was. I had to sit in the corner by myself, in a place that Clara said was cold and lonely, while she prepared wonderful food for herself and her mother. I was to listen to her rapturous descriptions of each wonderful dish, only to be told that I couldn't have any. This went on for the whole fifty minutes, while she repeated over and over again how bad I had been.

It seemed clear that Clara had intuited her mother's pregnancy, and I thought that the arrival of another baby might reassure her considerably after the miscarriage, which had happened so close to her own illness. However, the material about spilling suggested that her night terrors were the expression of primitive anxieties that were so overwhelming as to make ordinary developmental dependence impossible. We arranged that I should see Clara once a week, which was all that her parents felt they could manage. In fact, the therapy always felt precarious. Long holidays in her native country were one of the means by which Clara's mother coped with her husband's absences; the family culture made it hard for her to take on board the emotional impact on her daughter of missing sessions. While in other respects she was unfailingly reli-

able, I often felt as though I were a tyrannical figure whom she had
to placate, and I wondered about transgenerational issues. Clara's
extreme vulnerability made me feel a strong pressure to rearrange
my timetable in order to spare her the emotional consequences of
her parents' lifestyle.

The beginnings of therapy continued with the theme of me as
the bad child who was excluded from the marvellous meals, and
close intimacy being shared by a mother and baby. Clara's first
attempts to communicate her night-time fears suffered a severe
setback during a game when the father doll, infuriated at being
pushed out of the mother doll's bed by the baby, jumped up and
down so angrily on the double bed that it broke. This apparent
proof of the power of Clara's destructive wishes even after they
had been displaced onto the father doll put an end to any play
about night-time until I had found a more solid double bed. Until
then, she devoted herself to cooking games, producing food and
drink with plasticine and dirty painting water. I was supposed to
be very eager for these things, though their derivation from urine
and faeces became more and more obvious. However, when I
spoke very cautiously about how hard it might be not yet to be able
to produce food and babies, she encouraged me by saying, "Yes,
but I'll grow", and it was clear that she believed it. After this, her
cooking took on a different quality. She joined us up with string as
though by an umbilical cord, then tossed the tangled string on a
plate before offering it to me to eat. I said that it looked like spa-
ghetti, and she agreed. Apart from the fact that the umbilical cord
appeared to change from being a link between mother and baby to
being food under the mother's control, this was the first time that it
felt as though Clara were identified with a real mother whose
actions she had observed.

An important motif early in treatment concerned ways of maintaining contact without being joined by a string. Clara would go to
the lavatory whenever water got spilled in the sessions, as though
to reassure herself against the fear of spilling out of her own body.
She left the door open a crack: we could not see each other in
reality, but by moving on the lavatory seat she could control
whether or not our eyes met in the wall mirror. She played at
keeping in touch by speaking when we could not see each other,
and she liked to position herself so that she could see me in the

mirror without my seeing her. This variation on the cotton-reel game (Freud, 1920g) appeared to give her the necessary confidence to begin relinquishing the position of the adult. Instead of teaching me to write, she now asked me to write things for her: "Clara is drawing lovely pictures, and Charlotte comes and scratches her." Similar attacks on her skin seemed to underlie her night terrors— "monkeys come into the room at night and scratch me." Her sleeping improved dramatically following this material and the birth of her baby sister "Lisa", with whom she got on well. Jealousy towards the baby appeared to be largely contained in the sessions, as in her account of a nightmare: "Mummy went boom, then Lisa went boom, then there was a big thing that's frightening and a little hole that's frightening."

While work went ahead steadily during the body of the therapy term, any break threw Clara back onto being the adult, and I was not allowed to threaten this by having anything to say. "You're a chatterbox," she would say, which quickly rose to a shriek: " *Stop talking!*" After any gap in the treatment, she would scream this at me before she had got through the door. I experienced painfully just what it was like to be stripped of my capacities, which seemed to be so dangerous. Not long after her sister's birth, a crisis arose when Clara plucked covetously at my tights, asking whether they were what I was wearing. When I agreed, she said that she had tights too, but she soon insisted on knowing whether I had animals in my home. No attempt at interpretation would satisfy her, and her demands—which at the beginning had sounded controlling— became more and more desperate. It was as though I had to give up a way of working I believed in—my professional identity—or run the risk of traumatizing her (M. E. Rustin, 2001). Finally, she calmed down when I said that there was no need for us to tear things off each other, whether tights, animals, babies, or anything else—much as Anthony became able to share the ball in a game after I addressed his feeling that we were competing for one skin. She remained distressed for several weeks, but her mother continued to bring her when I explained that this was an important phase that was probably related to the miscarriages. After these crucial sessions, Clara was increasingly able to work on her own aggressive impulses without fearing a catastrophe. She informed me that she had no intention of clearing up—that was my job (and I agreed with her). She showed me her nails, threatening to scratch my skin, instead of seeing herself as the victim. We heard more and more about the Enormous Crocodile (a character in a children's book) who, as she said with relish, "eats babies", and her parents reported that she was eating enthusiastically, having previously always returned home from school with her lunchbox still full.

Not long before her fifth birthday, Clara enveloped us both in a big circle of string, then took it off and twisted it in the middle so that there were two loops joined at the centre. She placed one loop over each of our heads, though we remained joined in the middle. The following session, she cut the big loop in two and made a separate encircling boundary for each of us. We had each been given our own skin and our own identity. She now hardly ever brought her transitional object, which, significantly, was a piece of clothing from a baby doll which she used to hold against her cheek to help her to sleep.

Now that Clara no longer had troublesome symptoms, it became increasingly clear how intolerable her mother found the treatment. To avoid the therapy being broken off without a planned ending, we set a finishing date that was earlier than I would have wished. After a final therapy term dominated by oedipal rivalry towards both mother and father, I was left feeling that I had not been sufficiently able to defend Clara's vulnerability. Although her parents were happy with the results of treatment, I could imagine that Clara might protect herself by becoming a professional breaker of hearts in adolescence.

Discussion

Trauma, by definition, involves a piercing of the skin, whether physical or psychic. Against the background of her parents' attitude to loss and dependency, Clara had suffered a series of circumstances—being a replacement child, her father's prolonged absences, the move to London and its effect on her parents, her mother's second miscarriage, and Clara's own hospitalization—which, taken together, left her in a state of confusion. External events unhelpfully confirmed the destructive power of normal infantile aggressive impulses against parents and siblings (Cecchi, 1990), and the near-simultaneity of the move to London, her mother's miscarriage, and her own critical illness would have made for confusion between her mother's depression, the death of a rival, and her own threatened death. It was as though the skin membrane between her and other people had become too permeable (Rhode, 2000), leading to the fear that the external world was a reflection of her own fantasies, which were therefore too dangerous to own.

Two processes were central in the early stages of treatment: Clara's control of eye contact in the lavatory mirror, and her projection into me for containment of feelings of exclusion, badness, helplessness, and guilt. These processes made it possible gradually for her to assume her own skin and her own identity instead of competing with me for mine. However, breaks in the therapy seem to have been experienced as though I were stripping her of something essential, as in Tustin's description of competition for the bodily bit that ensures survival (Tustin, 1972)—in Clara's case, my words, the "skin" of my tights, and the animals/babies I was supposed to have at home. Her lack of a skin of her own seemed related to my possession of words, as though these words were both a means of projecting pain into her and also a sign that I was claiming the skin that should be hers. Young (1996) has described a patient with an eating disorder who similarly begged her not to talk, saying that he experienced her words on his skin as though on an open wound. The parallel is striking with baby Rachel, where the loss of the nipple is equated with an intrusive spoon, leading to an attack on the mother's skin barrier and, by identification with it, to Rachel's eczema; it must also be important that Clara's experience of uncontainable trauma took place before she could speak, and it was literally "lost for words".

Finally, I wish to highlight the skin function of Clara's transitional object. Winnicott writes: "*Of the transitional object it can be said that it is a matter of agreement between us and the baby that we will never ask the question 'Did you conceive of this or was it presented to you from without?' The important point is that no decision on this point is expected. The question is not to be formulated*" (Winnicott, 1951, pp. 239–240; italics in the original).

In fact, Clara's transitional object was   a piece of clothing belonging to a baby doll. To paraphrase Winnicott, the question it
allowed her not to be asked was whether the skin belonged to her
or to the babies who had not been born. When she held the piece of
clothing against her cheek, she could imagine that the "skin" belonged both to her and to the other babies, and she could get to
sleep without fear of monkeys scratching her. Tustin (1981a) has
described a similar experience of the confusion of ownership (as
distinct from sharing) which is characteristic of Bick's "adhesive
identification": when one leans against a chair, it can be difficult to
be sure what is the chair and what is one's own back. In Clara's
case, the use of the transitional object was based on adhesive phenomena. With the working through of her fears of destructiveness
and the strengthening of her sense of identity, the transitional object could be given up.

Conclusion

Clara's therapy made it possible to explore aspects of her catastrophic anxieties and to apprehend something of the issues concerning extreme vulnerability and life-or-death rivalries (Tustin,
1990) that played a part in her fundamentally loving relationship
with her mother. Esther Bick's insights into the foundations of the
sense of self are as central to understanding the symptom presented by a little girl with many obvious strengths as they are to
understanding children with autism or psychosis.

CHAPTER FOURTEEN

Failures to link:
attacks or defects,
disintegration or unintegration?

Anne Alvarez

E sther Bick was a superb clinician as well as a brilliant observer of infants. One of the many things she taught in the supervision on my first (five times weekly) case was the distinction between types of, and motives for, destructiveness. My little 4-year-old patient, "Laura", was a narcissistic and violently destructive child. She attacked me and the room relentlessly, often with great triumph and pleasure. One day the session started peacefully, with Laura painting. Suddenly, she noticed a small paint-stain on her spotless dress. She erupted once again with violence, which I linked with her usual furious impatience and intolerance of imperfection or frustration. Mrs Bick, however, suggested that at this moment it seemed to be more to do with unbearable guilt about damage. She saw the violence as escalating out of desperation as a result of a phantasy of an irreparable object, rather

An earlier version of this paper was published in the *Journal of Child Psychotherapy*, 24 (No. 2, 1998). I am grateful to Claudio Rotenberg, Giovanna Pasquali and Pia Massaglia for permission to use clinical and observational material.

than as a defence against persecutory frustration. And she stressed the escalation: the way the guilt could feed the violence and the violence the guilt. This was only one revelation among many, but it was typical. Her capacity to see the dark side of human nature and yet have compassion for its vulnerability and weakness was a great inspiration.

The above distinction between aggression as a defence against paranoid anxieties and that against depressive ones was, of course, already there in Kleinian theory (Klein, 1940): the distinction described below was not, and it brought a whole new dimension to the theory of splitting. Bick, in 1967, made the highly innovative distinction between "unintegration as a passive experience of total helplessness, and disintegration through splitting processes as an active defensive operation in the service of development" (Bick, 1968, p. 56 herein). She tied her theory so closely to the concept of the skin as the container of the unintegrated parts of the personality that the other ways in which she suggested that *the object facilitated integration* were hardly noticed. They were also somewhat superseded by the growing recognition of the importance of Bion's description of the maternal mental containing function, with its implications for the thinking mind and sanity (1962a). Yet it was left to Bick (and later, to Joan Symington in 1985) to explore the *consequences of the lack* of such maternal containment.

Reality, thinking, and learning

Both Bick's theory of containment, linked mostly with bodily holding, and Bion's, with mental holding, have spatial connotations. It may be useful, however, to explore the temporal elements in the move towards early integration, and the dynamic forms in which reality presents itself. I shall consider some of the ways in which single thoughts become thinkable and then look at the problem of links between thoughts—the problem set us by Bion in his great paper "Attacks on Linking" (1959). Bion takes what seem to be two rather contradictory positions regarding failures in links. One refers to the effect of destructive attacks on the patient's own ego and thinking; the other takes account of something more like a deficit in

linking (or what he might later have called an unrealized preconception of a link). The first seems to assume some prior development in the personality of a capacity to conceive of links or to make
links, followed by a destruction of this capacity. The second position describes the patient's inability or incapacity to think or to
store thoughts. At such moments Bion seems to be describing a
deficit in self or object or both, but at this point (1959) Bion did
not amplify on these remarks nor include them in his conclusion,
which concentrated only on the former position. However, Bick's
later careful distinction can inform our interpretive response to
our patients' problems of thought disorder and thinking deficit.
Clearly, the two positions need not be mutually contradictory: they
can coexist at the same moment in the same patient, but they
nonetheless need distinguishing. I shall conclude by indulging in
some speculation on possible connections between play that is
containing and integrating and the development of syntax.

Bion, like Freud (1911b), had stressed the importance of frustration for learning (1962b). He said that a preconception had to meet
with a realization for a conception to be born, but that a conception
had to meet with frustration for a thought to be born. He thought
that real learning depended on the choice between techniques for
evasion of reality and techniques for modification of it. I have
suggested that conceptions can be thoughts too and that the present
object in its aliveness and mobility may be as thought-provoking
and demanding of attention and interest as is the absent object
(Alvarez, 1988, 1999). Meltzer and Harris Williams, too, in discussing some babies' avoidance of the impact of passionate intimacy,
insist that "conflict about the present object is prior in significance to
the host of anxieties over the absent object" (Meltzer & Harris
Williams, 1988). I suggest that the present object possesses several
features important for the promotion of learning about reality:
its willingness to enliven, seek, and, when the child is depressed,
reclaim him; its eagerness to return to the child after absence, its
ability to receive pleasure and delight from the child, to permit
reparation, to forgive. Infant observation provides us with countless examples of these sorts of essential maternal functions: in one
observation, a little girl baby named "Lucy" had been prematurely
weaned and had become, in comparison to her usual sunny self,
somewhat depressed and withdrawn. During the observation, the

mother got down on her knees facing the baby, was tirelessly concerned and sympathetic, and gave far more of her face and voice on that day than on previous occasions when her breast had been available. This type of "cheering up" need not involve the kind of manic reassurance and denial of depression that could encourage the development of a false self in a child. The mother may have been demonstrating something different to her child: namely, her sympathetic understanding that although something was lost—the breast—not everything was lost, and that where there had seemed to be emptiness, there was still fullness and ripeness, after all.

The notion of the integrating features of a single present object can be extended to the oedipal situation, where the child is presented with two objects in a tripartite relationship that includes him and leaves room for all three. (See Abello & Perez-Sanchez, 1981, on the harmonious triangle which precedes the oedipal triangle.) Some links between two objects are made when the link between the two parents is seen as *for* the child—including the child, not excluding him—and their appearance together is timed or spaced sensitively, so that early integrations can take place.

The temporal form of reality: problems in having one thought

The cotton-reel game and the peekaboo game have been models for psychoanalytic theory about the absent object and about ways in which the infant comes to terms with reality: usually, as I have said, a reality of frustration, absence, and separation. There is, however, an equally primary reality—that is, the reality of the present object, but the present object realized in its dynamic shapes in time, its temporal forms. There are, as well as rhythmic comings and goings, rhythmic rockings, ebbs and flows. The present breast is sucked in bursts and pauses, in a basic rhythm of life which gradually gets regulated and can become as easy as breathing. Jerome Bruner has pointed out that the peekaboo game is preceded by something even earlier: a looming game, where mother plays with the distance between her face and her infant's face (Bruner &

Sherwood, 1976). Modulation and regulation of presence is a task for the infant that is probably prior to the one of maintaining object constancy throughout absence. Bartram has pointed out that it was crazy of her to have waited for her 2-year-old autistic patient to have said good-bye to his mother at the moment when he was having such an obviously difficult time processing the sudden arrival of his therapist (Bartram, 1999, p. 140). A good-bye implies some degree of internalization of a constant object, whereas many children with autism have great difficulty in taking in experience in the first place. Introjection is difficult enough for them, and surely introjection of experience has to precede a more durable internalization and representation. I shall offer the looming game and something musicians call the anacrusis—the suspenseful up-beat before the down-beat—as paradigms to be added to the cotton reel game and the peekaboo game. I have, I should say, found myself driven to attend to these microscopic or microanalytic levels through my difficulties in finding a way of lending meaning to the extremely fragmented and frenzied behaviour of a 4-year-old boy with severe autism, "Samuel", whom I discuss throughout this chapter.

Bion's concept of alpha function, the function of the mind that lends meaning to experience, suggests that the thought may have to be thinkable long before the therapist can or should concern him/herself with luxurious questions about who is having it (1962a). One thought at a time may be enough. But with Samuel and other more severely psychotic patients, even that consideration seems a luxury. There is hardly even a single thought on which to get a hold. I would not use Bion's term "debris" (1955), nor would I use Meltzer's concept of the "dismantled object" (1975), for both imply a prior intact structure. I would prefer to think of it as fleeting "*un*mantled" fragments. Samuel seemed to have been an unformed person in severely unintegrated states, who, even when he did emerge from his worst autism, did not know how to live in the time dimension. I had to start almost from scratch in helping Samuel to build a thought out of tiny strands. My problem was how to facilitate the links between the strands. After many months work, he did begin to take some more than fleeting interest in simple objects in his box, such as a little blue cube, and to explore them, but always only one at a time or in a bunch that was treated as a unit.

One game he chose was a "looming game" where he pulled me close and then pushed me away, or allowed his head to fall back so I could say, as in the more elaborate peekaboo for which he was not yet ready, "Where is Samuel? Oh, *there* he is!" Here, both self and object are provided with a modulating durability. This tiny expansion in time and of time began to extend to his play with objects in the room: in the beginning, he threw everything on the floor and never retrieved anything; he simply flitted to the next activity. I started by retrieving most things, but gradually I began to balance this with comments that he "really was still very interested in that yellow brick he had just thrown away, but he couldn't be bothered to pick it up". I insisted that we both knew he still really wanted it. He began to pick up many things and resume play with them. At a later stage, he finally began to try to conceive of twoness, but it nearly drove him mad. He and I had to learn that thinking two thoughts *takes time*, and time was something Samuel did not appear to have.

Bion on the relationships between thoughts

I think we owe to Bion the fact that we now have a psychoanalytic theory of the mind which corresponds to our subjective impressions: as well as a whole inner world full of living objects, memories, facts, and images, there are thoughts lit up by meaning and powered by their own energy. A mind is a vast panorama of thought-about feelings and felt-about thoughts, which are constantly in interaction with one another and with us. They are dynamic and energetic. Sometimes we succeed in putting two of them together, sometimes they get together on their own without our permission. Sometimes they haunt us, often they elude us.

In "Language and the Schizophrenic" (1955), Bion agreed with Freud that the psychotic patient is hostile to reality and that he also attacks his sense organs and his consciousness. Bion added that the psychotic patient attacks his capacity for verbal thought and that

this involved a very cruel and sadistic type of splitting. He continued throughout subsequent papers to alternate between descriptions of thought disorder that he ascribes to sadistic attacks and
others that he attributes to something more like ego deficit—rather
than a refusal to think, at times he is describing an inability to
think. He gives a dramatic example of active splitting, with a patient using language as a mode of action for the splitting of his
object (Bion, 1955) "The patient comes into the room, shakes me
warmly by the hand, and looking piercingly into my eyes says, 'I
think the sessions are not for a long while but stop me ever going
out'" (p. 226). Bion treats this material as the result of a piece of
active splitting. He acknowledges that the patient has a grievance
that the sessions are too few but interfere with his free time. He
takes it as an intentional split of the analyst to make him give two
interpretations at once. His evidence is that the patient goes on to
say, "How does the lift know what to do when I press two buttons
at once?"

Thanks to the later Bion (in   *Learning from Experience* , 1962a),
where he does have, as Grotstein (1981) has pointed out, a concept
of deficit in the containing object, I think we could try an alternative way of looking at the material: we could see this as a patient
who perhaps did not have enough ego or a sufficiently elastic
mental container to allow him to separate out those two thoughts.
The splitting may have been an urgent expression of two desperately pressing thoughts that arrived at once. The patient may have
felt he needed both to be understood at once, by a container that
could simultaneously take in both and gradually separate them out
for him—which is, in fact, what Bion did. Babies are often faced
with similar problems when they arrive at the breast too desperate
and frenzied to suck, hands thrashing about and blocking their
way to the nipple. The mother talks soothingly, moves the baby's
hands away gently, and helps the baby to find the nipple—that is,
one thing at a time, first this, then this, not both at once. Integration
(or what Bruner, 1968, calls coordination) depends on orderings of
both a spatial and a temporal kind, and before these can be internalized, these must first be provided by the object.

Bion does in fact take up the deficit issue on the next page: he
refers to the patient's difficulty in dreaming and in having phanta-

sies. He interprets to the patient that without dreams he has not got a way of thinking about his problem and later on (1962a, p. 236) says, "since you feel you lack words, you also feel you lack the means to store ideas in your mind". The patient said he couldn't remember what Bion had just said, and Bion replied, "this feeling is so strong it makes you think you have forgotten things". After this interpretation of the deficit, which, one can see, gave the patient his mind back, the patient was able to remember.

In the last example, Bion is addressing a general difficulty in thinking or dreaming—that is, in thinking any thought. In "Attacks on Linking" (1959), however, he goes further and examines failures to make, or to allow,   *links between* thoughts. He ascribes these failures as due to a destructive attack on the link between the creative couple, but the notion of a deficient capacity still comes in his interpretations to the patient. I think we owe to infant observation and infant development research the knowledge that there are times when the patient can really only afford to think one thought at a time. Not all couplings are creative. In a discussion of the development of the infant's capacity to coordinate sucking and looking into genuinely two-tracked thinking, Bruner, a cognitive psychologist, hypothesizes that this is the basis of the capacity for "thinking in parentheses" (1968). He stresses that this only arrives after the earlier stage where, in the early days of life, the child can only do one or the other, not both simultaneously. In spite of what I regard as Bion's overemphasis on attacked links, it is important to remember that his attention to the *emotional* significance of disturbances in links, to the emotionality that is intrinsic to thinking, and his later development of the concepts of alpha function and containment, were absolutely revolutionary and of course completely lacking in the cognitivists' descriptions of thinking.

Britton (1989) has introduced the concept of the "third position" for thinking: he suggested that where parental intercourse is felt to be too intrusive, the link between child and mother may be annihilated. He stressed the importance of the oedipal triangular space for thinking. In the cases described below, I shall be referring to deficits, not necessarily in space but in an inner sense of ordinal time, of sequentiality—that is, in a temporal container. These patients felt that they did not have time to think. My own patient,

Samuel, suffered from acute impatience, hatred, and greed within his own self, but this seemed to be accompanied by an impossibly transient and fleeting sense of an internal object that he experienced as never giving him time to find out about it, the links within it, and these links between it and other objects.

Clinical material

Samuel and twoness

When Samuel came into intensive treatment at the age of just 4 years, he had never played and had never shown any interest in toys or objects, other than to spin the wheels of little toy cars and thereby to get himself into an almost hypnotized state. Finally, he began, after about six months, to pick up two little cube-shaped blue bricks. He would look at them briefly, as though for a fleeting second he were examining and enjoying their sameness, their symmetry, and the way he could put the two together; then he would be overcome by excitement and agitation and would suddenly squash them together and explode them into the air. He would be overcome by the same sort of excitement whenever he came close and looked into my eyes or at my face. A further six months on, he slowed down a little and became able to study the shapes of the bricks closely, to build towers with them and add others, and to post some into appropriate holes in shape sorter toys. I wondered how this came about, and what may have been the major preconditions. I did not have the impression that the explosions were simply the result of an enraged attack on twoness. Samuel was having, I think, difficulty in coping with profound excitement and also with incomprehension. How could there be two of something, how could he look at two at once? He was having, I think, difficulty with the comprehension that twoness could be available to him *in time — that time would enable him to look at both, not necessarily at once. In fact, from the way he first began to look at my face, I got the impression he had never learned how to scan, which is how people look at eyes and faces.* In the beginning he never met my eyes for more than a peripheral fleeting instant, but, when he did, his gaze was too strong, and then he would have to tear his eyes away, just as babies do in the early days of life until they learn to scan (Stern, 1983). He needed a container that could help him to find out not only how to make do with one object or thought, but also how to have two, *in sequence*, one at a time. In fact, as he began to use his eyes more, and meet people's gazes from greater distances, his acute shortsightedness improved and his previously high glasses' prescription approached the normal. I guessed that he was finally using his eye muscles.

Bruner's research (1968) on how babies develop the capacity for two-tracked thinking and thinking in parentheses is of interest here: the babies move from one thought at a time where the second thought has to be excluded, on to alternation between the two, and finally to eventual coordination where one activity is soft-pedalled (in reserve) while the other is given foreground attention. In one infant observation of a baby called "Angela", we had already noted both her parents' sense of respect for their baby's agency and competence, but also for their own (Alvarez & Furgiuele, 1997). Already, in the mother's interaction with the baby, there were at least two figures in the picture, each with some recognizable space and competence of her own. Mother described how Angela, at 35 days, did not seem able to grasp the rattle on her own but could hold it if mother helped by putting it into her hand. At one point she said to Angela, "You like your friend the pendulum clock, don't you!", and then turned Angela so that she could see it better. At a feed in a later observation, mother showed some mild jealousy of the baby's seeming preference for her pendulum "friend" over finishing the first course of her meal, but she accepted defeat, did not insist that the baby finish, and offered some different, possibly more enticing food instead. A compromise offers a third option to two warring factions. A mother who waits while you express an interest in something else is remaining "in reserve" in a very significant way, and this is an emotional, but perhaps a cognitive experience too. At 4½ months mother remarked to the observer that Angela had begun to notice that she could pass something from one hand to the other! In fact, Angela became a very advanced baby and, as she approached the end of her first year, gave every sign that she could easily hold several thoughts in mind at once.

"Barbara" and fourness

A schizoid obsessional 13-year-old girl, Barbara, used to communicate in the most profoundly muddled way because all the thoughts emerged at once and seemed to be fighting for precedence. Barbara's language and learning improved considerably after some years of treatment. One day she said that the problem in the past was that she didn't dare make a thought wait, because she was certain she would lose it. If she had four things to say, her mind would jump ahead to numbers three and four, because they were demanding her attention, and then she would lose numbers one and two. Numbers three and four would never wait their turn in the queue, as it were, until she learned, somehow, both to tell them firmly to wait and to believe that they could and would. She seemed to have had an internal object that would not wait for her to get around to it, or back to it. Was Barbara's incoherence an attack on integration, or something to do with a need to have a container that could hold two or more thoughts in some sort of sequential and subordinating order? Although her own vast impatience played a part in the construction of these demanding internal objects, it is also true that when she began to see that they could wait, and could be made to wait, her cognition and verbal coherence improved dramatically.

"David" and the conjunctive link

David was a 19-year-old adolescent boy referred to a male psychotherapist for panic attacks and a total incapacity to write at school: every time he got to the end of a sentence, he felt it was dead and he could not go on. He was very withdrawn and obsessional, and probably hallucinating. By the time of this session, he had been in treatment for some months and was no longer hallucinating. He had begun to be able to write again, but with enormous difficulty.

This is the first session after the winter Christmas holiday:

> David comes five minutes late and gives an almost incoherent explanation. He then goes on to speak very fast about not being able to study. It is numbing, circular, and full of peculiar

rationalizations. He refers repetitively to knowledge getting lost and "falling in a hole", and he mentions briefly, before it gets lost in the circular talk, a wish to die. The therapist talks to him about a feeling of losing what he knows and that it feels like dying. The therapist also says that "When I go away it is like leaving him with a hole inside him where he loses, forgets the work we did in the past." The patient expresses some ambivalence but does slow down. Then the speed and circularity build up again, and the therapist, with great sensitivity, seems to enable him to slow down again. The patient says that he cannot write the word "and", he cannot write the word "the", and he cannot write "or". He uses hyphens instead. He says he is aware his essays are very long, so he cut those words and used the hyphens so as not to lose the meaning. The therapist says that he seems to feel that for meaning to exist there shouldn't be any link. David agrees and speeds up again, circling in search of meaning as though trying to get inside the text itself.

What is an "and"? It is a very special kind of link: it seems to contain a promise of more to come, not a death or a dead end. It ministers to one's greed and appetite but also to one's hope, expectation, anticipation, and perhaps also to one's fear and dread. In music, the suspenseful anacrusis, the up beat before the stressed down beat, also contains a promise. It builds up to the stressed beat, or the key word in the song, *Ta ra ra* BOOM *de ay*. Unlike my little autistic patient (Samuel), David was not completely out of touch with reality. He at least felt he had to offer some recognition—in the form of the hyphen—to the fact that nouns need link-words to join them with other nouns, and maybe somewhere to his need and desire for abbreviated waiting periods. He seems to feel that the links take too long, are endless. He wishes to shorten them, in the same way, perhaps, he would have liked to have shortened the winter break from his therapy. He wants a tighter, closer link. His difficulty with "the" may be because "the" may testify to the particularity and individuality of an internal mother or therapist. Perhaps specificity is a luxury when need is felt to be very urgent. David was in an acute panic about exams. How should we talk to such patients? What can they understand of our interpretations? Working with autistic children who have no language, one is always concerned to find the word, tone, or phrase that will most bestir mental activity and language, the word that will meet and match experience but expand it a little too. Sometimes a simple "Slow down, calm down, it's okay, there's enough time", or "It's okay, we are back together, the break is over", seems to help.

Samuel and the ordinal link: the "and" link in play

In the beginning, Samuel showed interest only in the flowing of water, the spinning of wheels, his own clenched hand, his reflection in any shiny surface he could find, and the occasional wild glance at me. Gradually, as he emerged from his frenzied states and showed more interest in me and in objects in the room, I introduced toys that I thought might be suitable for whatever extremely early developmental level might be being revealed in his non-autistic moments in the sessions. These children may give up autism, but tremendous developmental delay is usually revealed even in their newly normal moments. At one point, I provided a ring toy, a series of ever-larger brightly coloured plastic rings on a tapering pillar. Samuel loved it, but he hated the fact that the perfect shape could only be achieved by placing the rings on it in exactly the right sequence. He could just about tolerate a pile or a tower of the rings, but he loathed ordinal relations between things. His solution was to hurl the pillar away contemptuously and to build a tower of the rings in any order he chose, without using the pillar. He would, however, sometimes decide to build it properly, if I handed them to him in the right order, holding my breath and making suspenseful "and . . . the purple one, and . . . the blue one" before each one went on. I suppose what I was trying to do was to fill the previously intolerable gap with something that instead of threatening emptiness to this wildly impatient but also desperate little boy, contained a promise, but also a certain sort of teasing torment that was just bearable. This seemed to catch and harmonize with his own tortured inability to wait and to tolerate sequencing, but perhaps it also modified it and made it into a game—the beginning of anacrusis. Bion says the infant has to learn to modify reality, not to evade it, but I think that the implication of Bick's concept of unintegration is that reality also sometimes has to be modifiable and even to modify itself. Animate, living objects are constantly both self-modifying and being modified by the infant. The normal baby has experiences of reality as both unmodifiable and modifiable. This is not the place for a discussion of psycho-therapeutic technique with children with severe autism, but it is perhaps important to mention that Samuel's autism did seem to have been present in early infancy. His difficulties with attention span and eye contact, and his impatience with the otherness of the world, had, I suspect, left him closed to—and increasingly de-prived of—the ordinary modulating life experiences that enable cognitive and emotional development to go forward. Extreme ear-liness of onset can set the child on an ever more divergent path of development. Work with such severely autistic children thus needs to be developmentally as well as psychoanalytically informed: at times, a more active technique may be necessary where very early infantile deficits need addressing (Alvarez, 1996)

    After four years of psychotherapy, Samuel began to show real interest in three-person relationships, and real jealousy. He not only showed interest in slight changes in the room, or other people in the corridor of the clinic, he began to let me see his interest and, sometimes, even his outrage. I think, however, that his earlier dif-ficulties with links went deeper than an oedipal problem: micro-cosmic links—basic micro-integrations involved in the capacity to look and take in a mobile human face or to listen to a lullaby—may need to be established before larger oedipal links can be built.

Discussion: play and syntax

Is there a connection between syntactical link words such as "the" and "and" and "or" and very early play? Does the pre-language of play prepare infants for real speech and for the structure of real sentences? The teasing "and" is a link, a human one, which is free and playful. It also may be similar to what Bion would call an "articulated link". You don't exactly know *when* the ring will come, but you do know that it   *will* come, and in a way you do know when, because you can see it coming. The looming and receding object remains present. The alerting surprise comes in many forms, not always unpleasurable. Alfred Brendel (2001, p. 2) pointed out that Haydn surprised us with the unexpected, Mozart with the expected.

Sue Reid has referred to the difficulty that children with autism have in the "punctuation" of their experience. [1] This is something that Samuel was completely against—like the rests and pauses in music which are as important as the notes. If the patient thinks of pauses as an end of the world and of his mind, he dare not pause. Samuel eventually became able to look at bricks and also to pour the bricks from a large container to a smaller one. He began to enjoy the suspense about whether they would fall. Normal children love "Ready . . . steady . . . go!" games. Perhaps suspense is essential to language and is part of what we call prose style. Syntactical speech—structured sentences—unlike the telegraphic speech of the psychotic, involves some necessary capacity to tolerate suspense. Samuel began to use suspense less sadistically—he shared the joke instead. Experiences of bearable suspense, but more important, *games of suspense* that give symbolic meaning to such experience, may even have some connection with the origin of the subjunctive: what is the balance—between confidence in a secure world and fear of its untrustworthiness—that is necessary for doubt and hope to develop out of fear and manic denials? Instead of insisting on intrusive physical contact with me whenever he felt fond of me or in need of emotional contact, Samuel began to accept using a little chair beside me and, indeed, began to start every session by pulling it up towards me in expectation of a (proto-) conversation or some playful interaction. The taking and placing of the chair seemed to signal a belief in preparation and preludes and, more important, in the concept of a place and time for preparation and preludes. Instead of the need for desperate grabs at life, he seemed to be developing some idea of a waiting area and a waiting time that could be confidently expected to be followed by something worth preparing and waiting for.

The present object and the absent object—or the foreground object and the background object—are linked by the preparations for an entrance, the preparations for an exit. In musical terms, both

---

[1] Personal communication in 1994.

the anacrusis—the moment of suspense which nevertheless contains a promise—and the cadence that ends the phrase or musical piece are necessary to the form. What gets internalized in normal development is not just an object, or rather two objects, with spatial form, it is an object, or two objects, with a dynamic form: a shape in time. The link words, "the", "and", and "or" and Samuel's growing acceptance of, and even pleasure in, the rests and pauses in play may suggest something about the way in which the real human world gets internalized.

Do similar preludes help babies later to listen to "Once upon a time . . .", or "Well, then, what shall we do?" A "the" not only underlines the particularity of something, it warns us and prepares us for the fact that a *something* is coming. Articles and prepositions and verbs are link words but, like all links, contain a promise. Without that promise, links are inconceivable and waiting is a nightmare.

In conclusion, I suggest that Bick's concept of the need for early integration provides an important supplement to Freud's and Bion's ideas on how learning of reality takes place. Oedipal or oral frustrations and separation are all alerting experiences. But where disturbance is too great, thoughts may become unthinkable. Reality presents itself in temporal forms, which are the means by which presence and absence are linked, and also by which two presences are linked. The oedipal link, which excludes the child, may be not the only experience of an "and". Links between different versions of a present object have to be built alongside other more sophisticated ones concerning absent objects. The reel game and the peekaboo game have provided models for the absent object. The looming game or sequencing games may provide models for the modulating, integrating, object, which has a changing dynamic form in time but is not yet truly absent, just sometimes more and sometimes less within reach.

CHAPTER FIFTEEN

Looking in the right place: complexity theory, psychoanalysis, and infant observation

Michael Rustin

After over fifty years of the practice of Esther Bick's model of infant observation, there surely cannot be too much doubt about what is supposed to be observed in this setting. Esther Bick herself described the purposes of introducing infant observation into the curriculum of child psychotherapists as to "help the students to conceive vividly the infantile experience of their child patients" (1964, p. 37 herein). She refers also to "the student's understanding of the child's non-verbal behaviour" and to the student's "unique opportunity to observe the development of an infant more or less from birth, in his home setting and in his relation to his immediate family, and thus to find out for himself how these relations emerge" (p. 38 herein).

This is, in descriptive terms, clear enough, and it has been a good-enough guide to the educational purposes of infant observation. But when one thinks of infant observation as a resource for generating new ideas and understandings in psychoanalysis—that

An earlier version of this chapter was presented at a conference on "Origins and Evolution: The Interplay of Attachment Theory and British Object Relations", at the Under Fives' Study   Centre, University of Virginia, Charlottesville, 5–8 April 2001.

is, for research—it says rather little. For this purpose, a more theoretical discussion of the kinds of data and experience that infant
observation can provide, and how these relate to the development
of psychoanalytic theory, is necessary, as I have explored elsewhere (Rustin, 1989, 1997). In this chapter, drawing on the writings
of both Bick and Bion, I add some additional dimensions. I point to
some interesting parallels between the modelling and mapping
devices developed in recent work in complexity theory and chaos
theory (originating in mathematics, but now with broadening applications to empirical sciences), and psychoanalytic method and
then suggest how these are relevant to infant observation too. I
shall be suggesting that Bion and, in a more implicit way, Bick
anticipated by about twenty years the ways of thinking of complexity theory, but from their very different psychoanalytic starting
point.

There is an unavoidably abstract and meta-theoretical aspect to
these research questions, which involve the definition of our underlying objects of study. What kinds of meaning are we looking
for in clinical and observational studies? Are they the kinds of
regularities that are summarized in scientific laws, defining relations of cause and effect? Can they be generalized between instances? Can empirical evidence be found for such correlations as
we identify? Or are the links between observed phenomena merely
relations of logical coherence and consistency—what we think of as
the subjective meaning of an action or a state of mind, when we
understand how states of feeling, desire, and belief are connected
to one another? For example, we may understand an envious personality as one that is dominated by a pervasive (perhaps largely
unconscious) disposition or feeling, which gives meaning and coherence to various particular beliefs and actions of the subject.

Psychoanalytic explanation tends to waver between these different poles of cause and meaning. It needs the dimension of subjective and unconscious meaning to give any sense at all to its
work, but also it finds it difficult to do so without some idea of
causal connection or law-like relationship, to the discovery and
accumulation of which, of course, Freud was in particular dedi-
cated. Different research programmes in psychoanalysis and its
adjacent fields are shaped by these different polarities. The advo-
cates of "empirical research" in psychoanalysis seek to make psy-

choanalysis more compatible with "scientific" methods in which valid and reliable measures of causal relations are fundamental. Those committed, on the contrary, to clinical methods tend to stay closer to the dimensions of subjective meaning and to the individual case-studies in which these are most vividly manifested. The methodological difficulty for the latter is in finding systematic ways of generalizing from individual instances. The methodological difficulty for the former is to avoid, in their search for verifiable laws, such flattening out of individual differences and of the sheer complexity of psychic phenomena that they move far away from a psychoanalytic understanding.[1]

This polar opposition between dimensions of causality and meaning has long divided studies in the sciences—which once seemed to be unambiguously concerned with causality—from those in the humanities—which seemed largely concerned with meanings. The "human sciences" have sat uncomfortably in the middle of the division, some of them (such as psychology and economics) aiming to be as science-like as possible, while others, more preoccupied with dimensions of culture, such as anthropology and some branches of sociology, have given more weight to description—"thick description", as Clifford Geertz (1973) called it—over causal explanation, as the only way truthfully to render the complexity and contingency of human experience. Psychoanalysis has largely located itself on the subjective and meaningful end of this continuum. Kant's philosophical distinctions between the causally determined world of nature and the human domain of freedom and self-generated order have long provided an underlying metaphysical framing for this polarity of approaches.[2]

---

[1] Reflections on the relevance of complexity theory to the debate on evidence-based psychotherapy can be found in Robinson (2002). On the broader issues of evidence, see Rustin (2001b).

[2] The development of complexity theory, and its implications for psychoanalysis, match to some degree, however, Kant's own resolution of this antithesis, so far as human understanding is concerned, in his own account in   *The Critique of Judgement* of the order-creating capacities of the human mind. The post-Kleinian emphasis on the functions of mind and on the aesthetic sense as a manifestation of this has affinities with the argument of the *Critique of Judgement*, as both Likierman (1989) and Rustin (1991c) have pointed out in their discussions of psychoanalytic aesthetics.

The persistence and intractability of this opposition might suggest, however, that the problems have hitherto been framed in a misleading way. This seems especially suggested by the fact that, in the human sciences, both sides in this argument have often sought to overcome the limitations of their partial position by incorporating some of the insights of their antagonists. "Causal" approaches try to introduce a dimension of meaning—for example, by defining "meanings" and intentions as a particular kind of cause. Approaches focusing on meaning nevertheless identify developmental patterns, and self-maintaining "systems" or kinds of order, that seem to advance weak but unmistakable assertions of causal connection. Perhaps there might be another way of formulating the issues that can go beyond such pragmatic compromises between approaches into a more adequate formulation of what "binds" human actions together.

Complexity theory

I suggest we might find the more adequate formulations we need in the field of ideas known as "complexity theory" and "chaos theory" (Gell-Mann, 1994; Gleick, 1998; Kauffman, 1995; Prigogine, 1996; Prigogine & Stengers, 1984; Ruelle, 1991; Stewart, 1990), [3] which is just beginning to have a substantial impact on the human sciences (Byrne, 1998; Eve, Horsfall, & Lee, 1997; Thrift, 1999), and on the ways in which scientific explanations are framed. (For a useful overview of this field, see Taylor, 2001.)

---

[3] Chaos theory, developed initially by mathematicians and by physical scientists, sought to investigate unexpected properties of order in apparently chaotic or random environments. "Complexity theory" emerged subsequently from this, among scientists interested mainly in self-organizing biological systems. A literal and metaphorical boundary between these two overlapping frames of reference is the concept of "the edge of chaos". One hypothesis, developed through computer modelling of various evolutionary processes, is that the "edge of chaos" provides the optimal environment for development. "It is as though a position in the ordered regime near the transition to chaos affords the best mixture of stability and flexibility" (Kauffman, 1995, p. 91). Complexity theory became something of a social movement, its methodological holism, and its idea that order could be discerned in turbulent environments, giving a meta-theoretical backing to the idea of "sustainability". For a brief account of this social dimension, see Waldrop (1992, chapt. 9).

In the last twenty or so years, a major field of inquiry has developed around the significance in the natural, biological, and social sciences of complex self-organizing systems. The properties of these systems are not explicable or predictable by reference to models of linear causation. Of particular interest within this paradigm are changes from one ordered systemic state to another and the role of contingencies in bringing such changes about. They involve time-irreversible processes and are not neutral with respect to time as have been the models of both classical and quantum physics. They have the attribute that small changes in initial conditions can generate very large divergences in systemic outcomes (the famous "butterfly effect", in which the fluttering of the wings of a butterfly in the Amazon rain forest could in theory have major effects on a weather system in the United States). These systematic organizations show a tendency for "bifurcation", such that from a single starting point alternative structured outcomes are possible. Finally, there is a tendency for coherence and cohesion within such systems, which is explained by what are described in an extraordinarily resonant metaphor as "strange attractors".[4] "Strange attractors" describe the forces for cohesion and order in multidimensional systems whose states cannot be explained as the outcome of linear causal principles. One analogy used in this literature to make sense of "attractors" is that of neighbouring river basins, into one or other of which all the drainage of a locality must flow.

This paradigm identifies and explores a new kind of order, intermediate between the deterministic order of classical physics and the spheres of the apparently random and unpredictable. "Chaos", as defined within "chaos theory", is not chaos or randomness as this is understood in common-sense terms, but has its own different ordering principles, marked by major transitions, bifurcations of development, multidimensional causality, and "emergent properties", which are the outcome of interactions between entities within systems and of time-irreversible evolutionary patterns. The assumptions of constancy, determinism, and equilibrium, which

---

[4] Quinodoz (1997) writes that Ruelle, the originator of the "strange-attractor" concept, described his expression as "psychoanalytically suggestive". Indeed, what attractors could be stranger than those that are unconscious?

underlay previously conventional scientific paradigms, are replaced by the idea of evolution, partial uncertainty, and disequilibrium. The earlier assumptions (e.g. of classical physics) remain
valid within the assumption of "closed systems". However, it is
argued that the existence of closed systems cannot be presupposed.
(It is surely certain that human personality and social systems
never have the attributes of closed systems.) Quantum theory also
suggests that at micro-levels a principle of indeterminacy holds
(Heisenberg's "uncertainty principle" being one famous version of
this). This suggests that the actual world that we know through our
"coarse-grained" modelling is only one possible world of the many
that might have eventuated from the properties of nature. This is *a
fortiori* true of biological evolution and, of course, of the evolution
of culture and society, where there is no reason to presuppose a
law-like determination of one predestined present or future. [5] Psychoanalysis is predicated on the assumption that, for individuals,
different potential worlds can be imagined and realized, given self-
understanding. It is to make visible and possible such alternative
worlds that individuals enter psychotherapy.

This argument for necessary contingency does not depend, as in
some interpretations of quantum physics, on the uncertainties im-
parted by the place of the observer in any process of measurement.
(It is this idea that in science has linked the theory of relativity to the
idea of "relativism", or observation-dependent understanding. [6])

---

[5] Attempts, such as those of some forms of Marxism, to posit deterministic
laws of history have come to seem very fallible in contemporary "postmodern"
times.

[6] The psychoanalytic process involves complications of this kind, since
plainly the observed (the patient) is influenced by the process of observation
(by the analyst) in very substantial ways. For Grunbaum (1984, 1993) this
"observer-effect", or the suggestibility of the patient, is the fatal flaw in psychoanalytic claims to generate knowledge. Psychoanalytic method tries to deal
with this problem in various ways. Perhaps its most fundamental is the conten-
tion of object-relations theory that mental life is always organized in an ongoing
relationship to others, and that there could never be any way of apprehending
psychic reality which did not involve a relationship with an observer. The
psychoanalytic method takes specific account of this relationship, via the transference and countertransference. It thus becomes an explicit dimension of the
description and explanation of the phenomena being observed, not an unno-
ticed distortion of what would otherwise be an "objective" account.

Instead, uncertainty and unpredictability is deemed to be an attribute of reality itself (Gell-Mann, 1994; Prigogine, 1996). Organisms—and complex organisms like human life in particular—exhibit these states of unpredictability, emergent properties, and the common "bifurcation" of evolutionary paths, to an even greater degree than the physical universe, although within the framing of chaos theory they are in this respect continuous with and not a departure from the properties of the physical world. The patterns of different evolutionary pathways, generating "fitness landscapes" in which certain species evolve to dominate particular niches at the cost of reducing their evolutionary potential to occupy any other vacant ecological spaces, is an example of such systemic, contingent, and time-irreversible patterns. (The specialization of male peacocks in the elaboration of plumage for sexual display has, for example, cut off the potential of this species to evolve its capacities in other prospectively competitive attributes such as speed of flight or invisibility to predators.)

Complexity theory and psychoanalysis

Valuables articles by Moran (1991), Quinodoz (1997), and Miller (1999) have previously explored the relevance of chaos and complexity theory to psychoanalysis. These writers have argued that the domain of psychoanalysis is the investigation of the attributes of self-ordering multidimensional systems, not of the search for linear causal correlations between specified variables. There are a number of respects in which the theoretical framework generated within this paradigm provides a better fit with the models of the mind that psychoanalysis produces than theories that presuppose linear determinism. The idea of "phase changes" between different states of equilibrium, which may be triggered unpredictably by contingencies and which involve bifurcated developments between alternative patterns of order, meshes well with contemporary psychoanalytic theory. The concept of "strange attractors" as the organizing principles of coherent configurations of mind seems, in the view of these writers, also to be a potent one.

Thus, chaos theory or complexity theory seem to offer an invaluable means of escape from the unsatisfactory choice that psychoanalysis has long seemed to face between "causal" and deterministic models on the one hand, derived from Freud's aspirations to scientificity, and "hermeneutic" and "interpretative" schemas on the other. The former recognizes and seeks out relations of causality without which psychoanalysis would lack a theory of purposeful change or agency. But causal models of the classical kind have great difficulties in accounting for the complexity and multidimensionality of emotional and thinking processes as the essence of psychic structure and process. To be usefully applicable to mental life, the principle of causality needs to be somewhat dissociated from the idea of mechanism and determinism. Hermeneutic approaches, on the other hand, have the advantage that they enable analysts to follow and monitor the systems of meaning and intention, conscious and unconscious, that constitute the mental activities of their subjects. These models recognize complexity and ambiguity as essential attributes of mind and can take account of the ways in which changes in mental process and function take place in ways that are only partially constrained by, or logically inferable from, previous structures of meaning. They allow for the emergent properties of the mind, and for the many unforeseeable connections that it makes, even if a principled disavowal of causality rules out too much. Devoted to the explication of meanings as it must be, psychoanalysis also needs conceptions both of the constraining powers of structures of mind and of the causal efficacy of the analytic process in bringing about specifiable changes in the structures of the mind. It would be gravely impoverished without these.

What complexity theory suggests is that we can transcend this unwelcome dichotomy between causal reductionism on the one hand, and a merely interpretative investigation of narratives on the other. It suggests that we should be looking for order and coherence in a different place, neither in the spheres of intention and meaning alone, nor in the sphere of deterministic structures or "mechanisms", as they have sometimes been metaphorically called. Instead, this emergent paradigm suggests that we should be looking for ordering patterns of psychic coherence, functioning within specified parameters, and for sometimes sudden changes in state, often of a binary or bifurcated kind, triggered or catalysed by external or internal factors.

Quinodoz (1997) utilizes the idea of "tuning variables" derived from chaos theory to explain how multidimensional systems can evolve in response to specific factors. He suggests that the intensity of a "containing relationship" between infant and parents, or the intensity of a transference relationship within a personal analysis, can function as "tuning variables" enabling development to take place along a continuum—or, rather, by means of step-jumps—from modes of mental functioning with fewer "dimensions" to those with more.

British psychoanalytic thinking post-Bion has given a lot of importance to "three dimensionality" as a criterion of psychic development. In recent work (e.g. Britton, 1998a), the resolution of oedipal anxiety into the acceptance of three (or more) person relationships has been defined as a key index of psychic growth. But in reflecting on the nature of autism and post-autistic states and in seeking to understand the development of severely deprived children, this tradition has also attached importance to the incorporation of the realities of time, space, and causality into the understandings of the mind, as preconditions for its development. The reflexive recognition of "inner" mental space, in the self and in others, is a third aspect of dimensionality which is now given importance in the psychoanalytic theory of development.

While containing relationships can be understood as "benign" tuning variables, we can conversely view high levels of anxiety or deprivation as "negative" tuning variables. Where the former may support phase transitions from paranoid-schizoid to depressive modes of function (which, as Quinodoz points out, involves a move from fewer to more dimensions of complexity), the latter may induce shifts back towards the paranoid-schizoid end of the spectrum, with its simplified binary ordering of good and bad by mechanisms of splitting. Such high levels of psychic anxiety may be produced in populations by civil conflicts or by sudden economic insecurities and may, in their turn, give rise to persecutory kinds of behaviour.

An obvious convergence between chaos and complexity theory and psychoanalysis lies in Bion's concept of catastrophic change. Within the terms of complexity theory, we can say that Bion's concept describes "phase changes" from one state of psychic order to another potential state, providing a powerful example of the

ideas of disequilibrium and changes in phase-space that achieved
their broader currency through public dissemination of chaos
theory and complexity considerably later. Bion's attention seems to
have been drawn to Poincaré around the same time as the mathematicians who were developing chaos theory were beginning
their work, but well before this work became widely known. The
interest of complexity theorists in the critical importance of the
"edge of chaos" as a state from which development and complexity
arises is closely parallel to the importance and necessity of "catastrophic change" in Bion's view of the mind. [7]

Recent developments in the theory of transitions and oscillations between paranoid-schizoid, borderline, and depressive
modes of functioning appear to be usefully framed within these
notions of complex forms of order and evolution. Britton's (1998a)
recent theorizations of movements and oscillations between successive constellations of paranoid-schizoid and depressive functioning, each reorganizing and re-framing the phenomenological
contents of the temporally preceding phase in new ways, is valuable in its introduction of a temporal dimension into the idea of
psychic development. One might say that the implicit aspiration of
classical Kleinian theory was to devise models of the paranoid-
schizoid and depressive positions which were in principle "time-
reversible". They were, that is to say, such logically consistent and
closed models that it would be possible to imagine a mind ordered
by either the one principle of organization or the other and moving
backwards and forwards between them rather as one can imagine
a change of physical state from liquid to gaseous and back again.
What Bion's and subsequently Britton's formulations do is to add
to this account a necessarily temporal dimension, acknowledging
that each "cycle" of oscillations may and indeed must be different
from its predecessor in that it has to incorporate and process the
psychic experiences of the previous stage. At least, in a developing

---

[7] Another framing of these issues, termed "catastrophe theory", arose from
the work of the French mathematician René Thom (1975). This also gave rise to
a research programme with many applications (Woodcock & Davis, 1980; Zeeman, 1977), but seems to have run out of steam. The largely U.S.-based programme of development of chaos and complexity theories appears to have
found greater momentum, as well as a great deal of visibility, through popular
scientific writing.

mind this will happen; no doubt there are many clinical instances where there appears to be disappointingly little development, either out of the paranoid-schizoid position or even within each oscillation between paranoid-schizoid and depressive modes. But Britton's discussion of the life and work of a number of major writers (Milton, Blake, Wordsworth, Rilke) shows how this element of irreversible evolution can be seen in psychic development, whatever its ultimate outcome, and can be the primary psychic subject of an artist's work. [8]

Another concept in chaos theory that may have its place in psychoanalytic thinking is the idea of the "fractal": the idea that the patterns of order that make up complex systems, bound together by "strange attractors", may be found at all or at least many levels of a system, from the micro to the macro, and from elements of short duration to elements that persist over time. [9] The analysis of clinical cases over time may disclose movements between paranoid-schizoid, borderline, and depressive states of mind and the triggering factors that bring such movements about. Such "state changes" can be understood by reference to the progress or otherwise of a whole process of psychoanalytic psychotherapy, in terms of the differences between patients' states of mind at its beginning and end. But they may also be related to the meanings of beginnings and endings for patients within more circumscribed time-intervals within a process of psychotherapy, whether these intervals be bounded by holidays, by weekend breaks, or by the beginning and end of a single session. The idea is that what is constituted by a "paranoid-schizoid" or "depressive" form of psychic organization can be identified at each of these different levels

---

[8] There are other links to time that are important in psychotherapeutic work. One is the discovery that psychic damage and trauma can be transmitted across a generation to children, even when individuals in the parental (or grandparental) generation who were directly traumatized seem themselves to have survived. Selma Fraiberg's concept of the "ghost in the nursery" (Fraiberg, Adelson, & Shapiro, 1975) is one of the most influential formulations of this idea. Another, more benign instance is the "sleeper effect" described by Israel Kolvin—the evidence that long-term benefit may be obtained from psychoanalytic psychotherapy even when its short-term effects seem to have been small (Bell, Lyne, & Kolvin, 1989; Kolvin et al., 1988).

[9] The seminal work on fractals is *The Fractal Geometry of Nature*, by Benoit B. Mandelbrot (1977). See also Stewart (1989).

and scales. It is in this sense a "fractal", an organizing pattern that manifests itself "all the way down" within a psychoanalytic process, and in the patterns of mind of a patient that this illuminates.

Why should there be "strange attractors", systemic forms of organization, and irreversible evolutionary patterns in the psychic organizations theorized by psychoanalysis? In fact, theory in psychoanalysis is largely organized around such models. Freud's "stage" model of oral, anal, and genital development was one early version of these. The Kleinian binary model of the paranoid-schizoid and the depressive positions is another, to which has more recently been added a third intermediary term: borderline states. Freud's classifications of neurotic pathology, Kleinian descriptions of oscillations between loving and destructive states of mind, and Rosenfeld's and Meltzer's related models of narcissistic character structure are among the many examples one could give of such systemic structures, or "organizations", as Steiner (1993) explicitly calls them in referring to "pathological organizations".

Such models might have emerged merely in response to the subjective and heuristic need for coherence and simplification of complexity of practising analysts, rather than as reflections of the objective properties of their human subjects, but this seems unlikely. The reason why we posit a finite number of clearly defined "ideal types" of psychic organization, rather than assuming that psychic characteristics are evenly distributed along continua with no special clustering around "extreme" or "pure" types, is more likely to be because this is an accurate representation of psychic realities. (Gell-Mann, 1994, discusses "power laws" that map various kinds of naturally occurring distributions that suggest that regularities are a property of nature, not merely impositions by our own cognitive apparatus.) But if this is so in respect of psychic life, what are the ordering principles or "strange attractors" that make it so?

A functional need for coherence of perception and psychic organization, to simplify and make manageable the task of processing experience and making judgements about the world (in particular, the world of other human beings), is what seems to explain the persistence of distinct patterns of psychic organization. Symptoms, as Freud and many others have pointed out, are effective in concentrating anxiety on specific objects. They may displace

anxieties from their "real" objects to other spheres where unconscious fears, though paralysing, are nevertheless contained by the
symptom in some way. Paranoid-schizoid ways of viewing the
world define the good and the bad in unambiguous terms and
eliminate confusing uncertainty and doubt. Fight–flight can be a
viable strategy of self-defence, which is why individuals and communities default to it when anxiety levels become high. Depressive
anxieties, which involve recognition of the existence of the other
and concern for their well-being, demand the toleration of more
complex realities and a measure of trust in the environment as not
wholly retaliatory.

This "depressive" structure requires support from both external and internal realities, and where these are lacking or weakened
it will collapse. [10] We can think of the perception of external risk,
and the susceptibility to internally generated anxieties, as different
kinds of (interacting) "strange attractors" in forming paranoid-
schizoid structures of mind. It is the need to contain anxiety in
some definite and unambiguous form which seems to be the
common principle that determines that psychic organizations tend
towards coherence, and bifurcate around different forms of coherence. Another way of putting this is to say that the coherence that
analysts need to make sense of their task is also a functional need of
their subjects and, indeed, of all human mentality. This "strange
attractor"—the principle of psychic coherence itself—is a universal, a kind of internal psychic gravitation or frictional drag, ensur-
ing that psychic systems move in step-jumps from one form of
equilibrium to another and that their elements are rarely arrayed
in random disorder. [11]

The conceptions of an immanent tendency to order that are
found within psychoanalysis are congruent with the more general-

---

[10] Wendy Hollway and Tony Jefferson's (2000) work on citizens' fear of
crime valuably demonstrated that "internal" realities (unconscious anxieties)
were important in determining the extent of fear, independently of the external
"statistical" risks to which individuals were subject.

[11] Nor is random disorder as common a feature of physical nature as might
be supposed. For example, pebbles on the beach, which one might think of as
randomly located, are in fact sorted by the waves and tides according to their
weight and volume and are smoothed into rounded shapes by the force of
friction.

ized conceptions of complexity and chaos theory. What is more astonishing, however, is the explicit anticipation of these ideas in the work of Bion, twenty years before the publication of most of the key modern writings in this field. In   *Learning from Experience* (1962a), Bion quotes at length from Henri Poincaré [1854–1912], the mathematician who is now widely regarded as the originator of complexity theory:

> H. Poincaré describes the process of creation of a mathematical formulation thus:
>
> "If a new result is to have any value, it must unite elements long since known, but till then scattered and seemingly foreign to each other, and suddenly introduce order where the appearance of disorder reigned. Then it enables us to see at a glance each of these elements in the place it occupies as a whole. Not only is the new fact valuable on its own account, but it alone gives value to the old facts it unites. Our mind is as frail as our senses are; it would lose itself in the complexity of the world if that complexity were not harmonious; like the short-sighted, it would only see the details, and would be obliged to forget each of these details before examining the next, because it would be incapable of taking in the whole. The only facts worthy of our attention are those which introduce order into this complexity and so make it accessible to us" (Poincaré, 1908). [Bion, 1962a, p. 72]

Bion derives his concept of the "selected fact" from Poincaré's insight. Bion put it thus:

> I have used the term "selected fact" to describe that which the psycho-analyst must experience in the process of synthesis. The name of one element is used to particularise the selected fact, that is to say the name of that element in the realisation which appears to link together elements not hitherto seen to be connected. . . . The selected fact is the name of an emotional experience, the emotional experience of a sense of discovery of coherence. [1962a, p. 72]

Bion is here arguing for the primacy of experience of psychic reality over deductive law-like formulations, arguing that the latter can only be made once links have been made in the mind ("epistemological" links) between experienced phenomena. He suggests that Poincaré's description of finding harmonious order in complexity "closely resembles the psycho-analytical theory of paranoid-schizoid and depressive positions adumbrated by Mrs Klein" (p. 72).

This text of Bion's was of course central to his own reorientation of psychoanalysis towards the primacy within it of imaginative experience, which, he said, called for "negative capability" (Keats) as the precondition of understanding. Meltzer's subsequent characterizations of the aesthetic aspects of mental function developed from this idea. Bion, of course, also remained committed to the relevance of logical deductive systems and categorizations. However, he thought that these followed from a prior "emotional experience" of finding coherence in disordered and fragmented states and could not precede it. His concept of catastrophic change, as we have said, directly mirrors the concepts of changes of state that are elaborated within chaos theory and are there given mathematical formulations that seem unlikely to be achievable within the "open systems" of the mind.

It is noteworthy that the mathematical aspirations of Bion's work that probably aroused most scepticism among many psychoanalysts, and have been most difficult for them to follow up, were in fact responsible for his anticipation of this new and valuable framing of scientific understanding. Psychoanalysis has been sustained throughout by such links (sometimes, like this one, unexpected ones) with different fields of inquiry. Indeed such conjunctions may embody the kind of creative catastrophic change that Bion's psychoanalytic theory predicts and prescribes as essential to development.

Bion's concept of "selected fact" was later taken up by Edna O'Shaughnessy and other analysts [12] in the elaboration of the idea of the specifically "clinical fact" of the psychoanalytic session. This, in O'Shaughnessy's paper (1994), refers to a perception of the reality of the transference relationship at a given moment which can be successfully communicated to the patient. When a clinical fact has been correctly apprehended, it is not only the analyst but also the analysand who has this experience of perceiving an unexpected

---

[12] See the special 75th Anniversary Issue of the *International Journal of Psycho-Analysis*, 75 (1994) on "The Conceptualisation and Communication of Clinical Facts in Psychoanalysis".

coherence and meaning. This possibility of shared understanding is, of course, essential to the psychoanalytic process and develops Strachey's (1934) earlier idea of "mutative interpretation". This is one aspect of the way in which Bion's early anticipation of the insights of complexity theory has informed contemporary psychoanalytic thinking.[13]

The relevance of complexity theory to infant observation

What the above argument suggests is that researchers in psychoanalytic infant observation should be looking primarily not for causal correlations or sequences of linear development, but for ordering patterns, for the evidence of emergent systemic organization in the minds of infants and in the relationships between infants and those around them. There may be a good fit between the frame of inquiry set out by complexity theory and the procedures and techniques of "naturalistic" infant observation, just as there has been shown to be such a fit with the procedures of clinical research. What characterizes infant observation is a holistic approach, an open-mindedness in regard to internal and external aspects of the experience of infants and their families, and an interest in mapping changes and development over time, which is expressed in its predominantly narrative, case-study approach. What may be captured through these methods is a recognition of multidimensional patterns of organization (for example, the effects of a supportive or non-supportive presence of grandparents, or of a persecuting or benign internal mother); the identification of discrete "changes of state" or shifts of equilibria, sometimes through

---

[13] There is a reflexive aspect to the apparent correspondence between the theoretical self-organizing systems posited in modern psychoanalytic theory (the "pathological organizations" of Steiner, for example) and complexity theory. On the one hand, psychic structures do have this character. On the other hand, those psychic structures which have been categorized and defined in post-Kleinian psychoanalysis in particular have been deeply influenced by a psychoanalyst, namely Bion, who grasped the essence of chaos and complexity before this paradigm acquired a name, and have thus already been shaped by this way of thinking.

an observed crisis in relationships or in the observational setting; or the role of "tuning variables" of a benign form of containment, or its absence, in the psychic development of the infant. Researchers in infant observation need to clarify and systematize both the "structures" and "patterns" that can be established as norms for their observations and the observable "indicators" that tell them about the existence or strength of each such pattern.

Much of the literature on psychoanalytic infant observation describes exactly these forms of discovery. One of the innate principles of complexity theory—namely, the idea that there is an inherent tendency to order in apparently random phenomena—is fundamental to Bick's approach to the mind of the infant. She posited a need for the binding together of the self and its bodily and mental experiences as a primordial psychic fact. The principal function of maternal containment is to support this sense of coherence and to protect the infant against anxieties of "falling to pieces". Bick's most important substantive discovery, her theory of the "second skin" (1968), has this primordial anxiety as its backdrop:

> The thesis is that in its most primitive form the parts of the personality are felt to have no binding force among themselves and must therefore be held together in a way that is experienced by them passively, by the skin functioning as a boundary. But this internal function of containing the parts of the self is dependent initially on the introjection of an external object, experienced as capable of fulfilling this function. Later, identification with this function of the object supersedes the unintegrated state and gives rise to the fantasy of internal and external spaces. [1968, pp. 55–56 herein]

Bick went on to describe how

> The need for a containing object would seem, in the infantile unintegrated state, to produce a frantic search for an object—a light, a voice, a smell, or other sensual object—which can hold the attention and thereby be experienced, momentarily at least, as holding the parts of the personality together. The optimal object is the nipple in the mouth, together with the holding and talking and familiar smelling mother.
> Material will show how this containing object is experienced concretely as a skin. Faulty development of this primal skin

function can be seen to result either from defects in the adequacy of the actual object or from fantasy attacks on it, which impair introjection. Disturbance in the primal skin function can lead to a development of a "second-skin" formation through which dependence on the object is replaced by a pseudo-independence, by the inappropriate use of certain mental functions, or perhaps innate talents, for the purpose of creating a substitute for this skin container function. [1968, p. 56 herein]

In one of the seminal psychoanalytic contributions to the infant's psychic development, she defined this, drawing on infant observational case examples, as the "second-skin" formation (Bick, 1968).

In her essay "Notes on Infant Observation in Psycho-Analytic Training" (1964), Bick makes frequent reference to the "patterns of behaviour" that are discerned in infants by observers. She describes these patterns in very concrete terms—for example, the different gestures of a baby's hands in relation to its mother's two breasts—and offers many conjectures on what these may signify in terms of psychic development. For example, in that particular case, that these different gestures suggest a kind of incipient splitting. The idea that "patterns" are what one should be looking for, whether in the minutiae of physical movements or in a broader mind–body configuration such as that of the "second skin", is an example of the kind of structure that one might expect to find in open self-organizing systems, especially but not exclusively in living forms, and in human subjects in particular. [14]

Many of the most fertile insights of infant observation research to date are of this kind. To the example of Bick's papers one could add many others, including Juliet Hopkins' (1996) article on the pattern and consequences for development of "too-good mothering" and the work of Sue Reid (1997) on observed patterns of mother–infant interaction that seem conducive to the development of autism. Another recent example of the identification of a "pattern" of this kind is in Pamela Sorensen's (2000) paper "Observations on Transition Facilitating Behaviour—Developmental and

---

[14] Once again, the convergence of Bick's ideas with the underlying conceptions of complexity theory, and with the ideas of Bion that anticipate these, was only to be expected. Bick refers to "situations conducive to catastrophic anxieties in the unintegrated state" in her second-skin paper presented in 1967 (published in 1968), indicating her closeness to Bion's thinking at that time.

Theoretical Implications". This paper, which is based on observations of the experiences of exceptionally vulnerable infants in a neo-natal intensive care unit and seeks to establish a bridge between attachment and object-relations theories, clarifies the importance of everyday transitions for all babies,. The exploration and elaboration of different forms of containment has become one of the principal areas of infant observational research (Briggs, 1997a). Along with a developing capacity to discriminate different patterns of containment, including those involving severe deficits or disturbances, have come the beginnings of purposefully "therapeutic" infant observations, where some measure of deliberate intervention takes place. This reflects a greater confidence in the ability of observers to understand from an early stage what is going on in an infant's relationships to those close to him. But, as in psychotherapy itself, the possibility of testing the outcome of interventions is likely to provide an additional resource for the development of new understandings and concepts.

Once theoretical classifications have become established as stable points of reference, they become capable of further differentiation—even "bifurcation", to use the terminology of complexity theory (as in the differentiation by Rosenfeld between libidinal and destructive narcissism). It is in this way that the adequacy and complexity of the theoretical models available for researchers can develop as they conduct observations.

The assumption of complexity theory that realities are complex, emergent, non-reversible over time, and liable to generate increased difference is consistent with both the humanistic and the scientific assumptions of psychoanalysis—humanistic, because psychoanalysis is committed to the inherent value of autonomy, difference, and choice (it wants its subjects to be understood and to understand themselves in their particularity, not merely as an instance of a diagnostic category); scientific, because the theoretical models of psychoanalysis have never been intended to do more than define the boundary conditions of different kind of mental and emotional life, within and between which much variation is both anticipated and desired.

The specific focus of psychoanalytic infant observation, conducted in natural settings, contrasts with the investigations of infant development undertaken within the "attachment theory" perspective, though their findings are in some respects mutually supportive. Attachment theory is wedded to a more classical scientific model, being committed to the identification of definite causal patterns or models of attachment and its preconditions. These models do capture some important boundary conditions that determine the capacity for relationships and well-being. In doing so, they identify temporal and relational spaces where developmental vulnerability lies and in which preventive interventions are feasible and desirable. But these approaches seem to have stopped short of much further differentiation, once they had established their basic array of framing conditions. (Three main kinds of attachment —securely-attached, anxious attached avoidant, anxious attached ambivalent / resistant—were discovered by Mary Ainsworth [Ainsworth et al., 1978], and a fourth—the disorganized / disoriented— was subsequently and valuably added by Mary Main [Main & Hesse, 1990; Main & Solomon, 1986].) This experimental methodology seems to have only limited conceptual resources with which to map either differences between individuals or their patterns of psychological development.[15] We could say, following Gell-Mann's (1994) term for broader interpretative schema, that these models are "coarse-grained" simplifications of realities that psychoanalysis and psychoanalytic infant observation seek to investigate in more "fine-grained" ways. The finer the grain of observation, the more that contingencies and differences become evident.

The increasing emphasis within the attachment-theory tradition on "mental models and maps" has increased the explanatory coherence of its models and brought it closer to psychoanalysis, in part through the incorporation of some of Bion's ideas. We could say that the capacity for the mental processing of experience is functioning within this paradigm as the "strange attractor" that holds its different patterns of attachment together. But it continues to lack the multidimensionality of the psychoanalytic theory of personality development. Psychoanalysis, it will be remembered, takes account of the dimensions contributed by predispositions to love and hate, as well as by the capacity for understanding, and by

---

[15] Peter Fonagy's comments on the challenges posed by psychoanalysis to attachment theory in chapter 13 of his *Attachment Theory and Psychoanalysis* (2001) are perceptive about their differences of approach.

the role of unconscious representations and memories internalized as phantasies of self and others. It seeks to investigate in its fine-grained way the idiosyncratic "scripts", both conscious and unconscious, that evolve as means of dealing with emotionally charged realities.

There is a natural continuum and complementarity between fine- and coarse-grained forms of explanation, and between the more conjectural and complex forms of explanation that go with the first and the more definite and categorical causal explanations that go with the second. One can say, therefore, that both clinical and observational psychoanalytic approaches, and protocol-driven and laboratory-based attachment-theory procedures, have their necessary and distinct place in the investigation of infant development (Rustin, 2001a).

What about the role of causality within these different models? Should psychoanalysis—and infant observation research in particular—be seeking to establish causal laws or not? In what way, if any, does the contribution of complexity theory resolve the antithesis between "interpretative" and "causal" models of explanation that we posited at the outset as a long-standing dilemma for psychoanalysis?

The identification of "patterns", "self-organizing systems", and "strange attractors" within complexity theory substitutes complex and holistic notions of causal relation for the "linear" models aspired to by many mechanistic sciences, including much of psychology. Complexity theory, and its applications within psychoanalysis, identifies "fields of force" that bind psychic phenomena and create or constitute dispositions for subjects to act according to discernible patterns. The paranoid-schizoid and depressive positions are examples of dispositions of this kind. These are "generative structures", [16] to use another terminology, with many

---

[16] The concept of "generative structures" derives from Roy Bhaskar's realist theory of science (Bhaskar, 1975). According to this view, theories identify and model structures that are manifested primarily through their observable effects. Scientific inquiry therefore involves not only making empirical observations, and finding correlations between them, but also making inferences from observed data to underlying structures and mechanisms. Reviews of this approach in relation to psychoanalysis are given in Will (1980, 1986) and Rustin (1991b). Psychoanalysis is distinctive in its assumption that surface manifesta-

connected dimensions. Their value for psychoanalysts, whether as clinicians or researchers, is not as predictors of specific acts, but as binding conceptions that specify tendencies or dispositions with many connected dimensions—for example, of thought, feeling, and behaviour. It *is* possible to identify typical causal connections within these theoretical schema and to find ways of accurately measuring the incidence of these. (Bick, for example, suggested that certain kinds of deficient containment would lead to defences of pseudo-independent "muscularity"; there is no reason to think that this could not be treated as a definite hypothesis and specifically tested against evidence.) But the interest and value of these models lies in their capacity to give definition to many differentiated kinds of pattern, as these appear in observational or clinical settings. This is why its preferred style of thinking is in terms of multidimensional narratives, rather than by the correlation of discrete variables. These models are not well adapted to demonstrating specific linear causal effects between identified variables, of the kind that evidence-based policy might wish to see. But they are powerful in identifying more holistic patterns of behaviour, and their antecedents and effects, and enabling skilled therapists to identify, within these patterns, areas in which change and development is possible.[17]

Psychoanalysis is antithetical in this respect to attachment theory, which gives much higher priority to the simplifications and

---

tions of consciousness and behaviour are derived causally from structures of mind that are held to be effective at "deep" levels of the mind, and whose existence and power has to be inferred from the "surface" phenomena of consciousness. Freud's theory of repression explained why these structures remained largely "unconscious". The idea of "mechanism" becomes important in psychoanalytic discourse through Anna Freud's theory (1936) of mechanisms of defence.

[17] Another model of explanation that is relevant here is the "part–whole" analysis, which is advocated by Thomas Scheff (1997) as often most appropriate in the human sciences. Where self-maintaining systems exist—for example, in biological organisms, or in social organizations or processes—the most useful form of explanation may be to clarify the relationship of specific phenomena to the larger structure and process of which they form part. "Catastrophic changes" from one pattern of systemic coherence to another create new part–whole relations, which then become a matter for investigation. Psychoanalytic interpretation often looks for connections of this kind. On the part–whole analysis of narrative texts, see Wengraf (2001).

generalizations necessary to establish robust causal connections (which, of course, it has done with success). The value of complexity theory for psychoanalysis is that it provides a much more adequate meta-framework for its ways of thinking than did the mechanistic models that have earlier dominated the sciences. There is a large domain of nature, it suggests, that is neither determined in the manner of a closed mechanism or system nor wholly random, indeterminate, or "free". Instead, it posits self-organizing systems, of high complexity, and indeterminacy within understood limits. This domain is precisely, in fact, the world of experience with which clinical psychoanalysts continually struggle and which observers encounter on a weekly basis in their visits to infants and their families.

In the forty years since the publication of T. S. Kuhn's *Structure of Scientific Revolutions* (1962), the recognition of the actual diversity and complexity of the sciences has made it easier for psychoanalysts to locate their work as having a place within a larger scientific community, the methods of psychoanalysis seeming less anomalous once these are understood as appropriate to their specific topics of study.[18] It seems likely that "complexity theory" offers a further illumination of this kind. It turns out that complexity, emergent properties, susceptibility to phase-transitions ("catastrophic change", in Bion's, 1965, 1970, terms), individual difference, and ubiquitous contingency may be normal facts of mental life, not merely the imprecise reflections of the inadequate scientific method of psychoanalysis. Not only are these complex and seemingly chaotic structures characteristic of the psychic realities that psychoanalysis investigates, but they seem now to have been found to be the attributes of a good part of biological and material nature besides.

---

[18] On the diversity of methods even in the natural sciences, see Galison and Stump (1996) and Knorr-Cetina (1999).

Endpiece

A s this collection of essays for her centenary clearly shows, Esther Bick's work has provided both a beacon and a foundation for her students and for those whom they in turn have trained in infant observation. Each contribution has been an example of a way in which her method and discoveries are now used and developed. In this they have given us a sight of the steadily growing bodies of experience and knowledge in the clinical, research, and teaching domains that are inspired by her work.

Before she introduced infant observation to the training of child psychotherapists and child analysts, trainees and candidates did not have such a rich opportunity to heighten their sensitivity to the whole observational setting. In attending to the importance of the observer's experience of the infant and family, and the way in which the role is both affected by and affects the setting, her method can be said to have made a tremendous contribution to the naturalistic, reflexive approach of both clinical and research psychoanalysis to their field of enquiry. This was part of her "stroke of genius", to requote Martha Harris. As an observational method that enables access to a reflexive understanding of the observer and the observed, it has much to contribute to the wider field of the social sciences, where there is a great need for such a sound qualitative methodology.

Bick had a passion fuelling her curiosity that lead to her making new discoveries, a passion with which her method is imbued. One can so often see in those who have been introduced to infant observation that their interest, too, has been ignited. The essays in this collection all show their authors' passion for Esther Bick's approach and thus extend her spirit that bit further in the domains to which she first drew us.

Bick's own use of her method allowed her to make the discoveries she reported and discussed in the two papers on the experience and function of the skin (1968, 1986). On first publication these were pioneering and highly creative—and they remain so today. It is often said by those whom she trained or supervised that Bick had a passion for discovering more about the emotional experience of the newborn and, particularly, his struggle for survival. This comes through very clearly in these two papers, which surely could not have been conceived without such a love for and curiosity about life as hers. This love, in turn, can easily be seen in the essays that have formed this festschrift. In each we see a different application or development of one or more of her ideas, whether they come from infant observation, the clinical papers, or both. In this, all the essays break new ground. Some take us further into the boundary between the sensual and the mental in the internal world of the infant, others explore responses to serious difficulties in the mother–infant relationship that give rise to drastic responses by the infant in the face of the grim necessity to survive, yet others explore ways of working clinically with children who have suffered such an experience. Along with these more clinically based contributions, there are those that explore other applications of infant observation. Some have introduced us to its power as a tool for assessing risk to children, others to it being a method underpinning and guiding a multidisciplinary-team-based approach to such a difficult and, sadly, increasingly common area of the child psychotherapist's work. There are also others that have shown how material as data from infant observation, in being especially clear about the actual experience of the child, is invaluable to court reports and research. This also supports claims that such a method is scientific and able to hold its ground with other research methodologies in use within the wider academic fora. It is, perhaps, no surprise that while one essay is devoted to discussing a highly innovative use of infant observation in the training of an allied profession, aspects of others have given us insight into such an important new development.

Psychoanalysis is a relatively new science and Bick's contribution is a relatively recent one. In this sense we have really only just begun to utilize the potential in her work for helping us to discover and understand new things about emotional life in human development. Thus it is enormously encouraging to note that child psychotherapists are currently being asked to meet an increased demand by a range of professions for training in infant observation. With this, and the international expansion of interest in her method that has been underway for some time, the future looks a very promising one for Esther Bick's work and spirit.

REFERENCES

Abello, N., & Perez-Sanchez, M. (1981). Concerning narcissism, homo-
sexuality, and Oedipus: clinical observations. *Revue Française de Psychanalyse, 45* (4): 767–775.

Ainsworth, M. D. S., Blehar, M. C., Waters, E., & Wall, S. (1978).
Patterns of Attachment: A Psychological Study of the Strange Situation.
Hillsdale, NJ: Erlbaum.

Alvarez, A. (1988). Beyond the unpleasure principle: some preconditions for thinking through play. *Journal of Child Psychotherapy, 14* (2).

Alvarez, A. (1992). *Live Company.* London & New York: Routledge.

Alvarez, A. (1996). Addressing the element of deficit in children with
autism: psychotherapy which is both psychoanalytically and
developmentally informed. *Clinical Child Psychology and Psychiatry, 1* (4).

Alvarez, A. (1999). Frustration and separateness, delight and connectedness: reflections on the conditions under which bad and
good surprises are conducive to learning. *Journal of Child Psychotherapy, 25* (2).

Alvarez, A., & Furgiuele, P. (1997). Speculations on the infant's sense
of agency: the sense of abundance and the capacity to think in

parentheses. In: S. Reid (Ed.), *Developments in Infant Observation: The Tavistock Model*. London: Routledge.

Anzieu, D. (1985). *Le Moi-Peau*. Paris: Dunod.

Anzieu, D. (Ed.) (1987). *Psychic Envelopes*. London: Karnac, 1990.

Anzieu, D. (1989). *The Skin Ego*. London: Yale.

Bartram, P. (1999). Sean: from solitary invulnerability to the beginnings of reciprocity at very early infantile levels. In: A. Alvarez & S. Reid (Eds.), *Autism and Personality: Findings from the Tavistock Autism Workshop*. London: Routledge.

Bell, V., Lyne S., & Kolvin, I. (1989). Play group therapy: processes, patterns and delayed effects. In: M. H. Schmidt & H. Remschidt (Eds.), *Needs and Prospects of Child and Adolescent Psychiatry*. Stuttgart: Hogrefe & Huber.

Bhaskar, R. (1975). *A Realist Theory of Science*. Leeds: Leeds Books.

Bick, E. (1962). Child analysis today. *International Journal of Psycho-Analysis, 43*. [*See chapter 2, this volume.*]

Bick, E. (1964). Notes on infant observation in psycho-analytic training. *International Journal of Psycho-Analysis, 45*. [*See chapter 1, this volume.*]

Bick, E. (1968). The experience of the skin in early object relations. *International Journal of Psycho-Analysis, 49*. [*See chapter 3, this volume.*]

Bick, E. (1986). Further considerations on the function of the skin in early object relations. *British Journal of Psychotherapy, 2* (4). [*See chapter 4, this volume.*]

Bick, E. (2001). Anxieties underlying phobia of sexual intercourse in a woman. *British Journal of Psychotherapy, 18* (1).

Bion, W. R. (1955). Language and the schizophrenic. In: M. Klein, P. Heimann, & R. E. Money-Kyrle (Eds.), *New Directions in Psycho-Analysis: The Significance of Infant Conflict in the Pattern of Adult Behaviour*. London: Tavistock.

Bion, W. R. (1959). Attacks on linking. In: *Second Thoughts: Selected Papers on Psycho-Analysis*. London: Heinemann, 1967.

Bion, W. R. (1962a). *Learning from Experience*. London: Heinemann. Reprinted London: Karnac, 1984.

Bion, W. R. (1962b). A theory of thinking. In: *Second Thoughts: Selected Papers on Psycho-Analysis*. London: Heinemann, 1967.

Bion, W. R. (1965). *Transformations*. London: Heinemann. Reprinted London: Karnac, 1984.

Bion, W. R. (1967). Notes on memory and desire. *Psychoanalytic Forum*, 2: 272–273, 279–280.

Bion, W. R. (1970). *Attention and Interpretation*. London: Heinemann. Reprinted London: Karnac, 1984.

Blake, P. (2001). Thinking outside, not inside: making interpretations hearable. In: J. Edwards (Ed.), *Being Alive*. London: Brunner-Routledge.

Bower, T. (1989). *The Rational Infant: Learning in Infancy*. New York: W. H. Freeman.

Brazelton, T., Koslowski, B., & Main, M. (1974). The origins of reciprocity: the early mother–infant interaction. In: M. Lewis & L. Rosenblum (Eds.), *The Effect of the Infant on Its Caregivers*. London: Wiley Interscience.

Brendel, A. (2001). *Alfred Brendel on Music: Collected Essays* . London: Robson Books.

Briggs, A. (forthcoming). *The Emergence of Child Psychotherapy as a Profession in Postwar Britain*.

Briggs, S. (1997a). *Growth and Risk in Infancy*. London: Jessica Kingsley.

Briggs, S. (1997b). Observing when infants are at potential risk. In: S. Reid (Ed.), *Developments in Infant Observation: The Tavistock Model*. London: Routledge.

Britton, R. (1989). The missing link: parental sexuality in the Oedipus complex. In: J. Steiner (Ed.), *The Oedipus Complex Today: Clinical Implications*. London: Karnac.

Britton, R. (1998a). *Belief and Imagination: Explorations in Psychoanalysis*. London: Routledge / Institute of Psychoanalysis.

Britton, R. (1998b). Naming and containing. In: *Belief and Imagination: Explorations in Psychoanalysis*. London: Routledge / Institute of Psychoanalysis.

Britton, R. (1998c). Subjectivity, objectivity and the triangular space. In: *Belief and Imagination: Explorations in Psychoanalysis*. London: Routledge / Institute of Psychoanalysis.

Britton, R. (1999). Discussion of Domenico and Giovanna Di Ceglie's paper: "Thoughts on Structure and Function of the Body in Symbol Formation." *Bulletin of the British Psychoanalytical Society*, 35 (7).

Bruner, J. S. (1968). *Processes of Cognitive Growth: Infancy* . Worcester, MA: Clark University Press.

Bruner, J. S., & Sherwood, V. (1976). Peekaboo and the learning of rule structures. In: J. S. Bruner et al., *Play—Its Role in Development and Evolution*. Harmondsworth: Penguin, 1985.

Byrne, D. (1998). *Complexity Theory and the Social Sciences: An Introduction*. London: Routledge.

Cecchi, V. (1990). The analysis of a little girl with an autistic syndrome. *International Journal of Psycho-Analysis, 71*: 403–410.

Coltart, N. (1986). "Slouching towards Bethlehem" . . . or thinking the unthinkable in psychoanalysis. In: G. Kohon (Ed.), *The British School of Psychoanalysis: The Independent Tradition*. London: Free Association Books.

Coote, S. (1995). *John Keats: A Life*. London: Hodder & Stoughton.

Cornwell, J. (1983). Crisis and survival in infancy. *Journal of Child Psychotherapy, 9* (1): 25–33.

Cornwell, J. (1985). The survival functions of primitive omnipotence, *International Journal of Psycho-Analysis, 66* (4): 481–489.

Di Ceglie, D., & Di Ceglie, G. R. (1999). Thoughts on structure and function of the body in symbol formation. *Bulletin of the British Psychoanalytical Society, 35* (7).

Donati, F. (1989). Madness and morale: a chronic psychiatric ward. In: R. D. Hinshelwood & W. Skogstad (Eds.), *Observing Organisations*. London: Routledge, 2000.

Dubinsky, A., & Bazhenova, O. (1997). Moments of discovery, times of learning. In: S. Reid (Ed.), *Developments in Infant Observation: The Tavistock Model*. London: Routledge.

Emanuel, R. (2001). A-void: an exploration of defences against sensing nothingness. *International Journal of Psycho-Analysis, 82*: 1069–1082.

Eve, R. A., Horsfall, S., & Lee, M. E. (Eds.) (1997).*Chaos, Complexity and Sociology*. London: Sage.

Ferenczi, S. (1933). Confusion of tongues between adults and the child. In: *Final Contributions to the Problems and Methods of Psycho-Analysis*. London: Hogarth Press, 1955.

Fonagy, P. (2001). *Attachment Theory and Psychoanalysis*. New York: Other Press.

Fraiberg, S. H., Adelson, E., & Shapiro, V. (1975). Ghosts in the nursery: a psychoanalytic approach to the problems of impaired infant–mother relationships. *Journal of the American Academy of Child Psychology, 14*: 387–422.

Freud, A. (1936).   *The Ego and the Mechanisms of Defence*   . London: Karnac, 1993.

Freud, A. (1951). Observations on child development. In: *The Writings of Anna Freud, Vol. 5* . New York: International Universities Press, 1969.

Freud, A. (1953). Some remarks on infant observation.   *Psychoanalytic Study of the Child, 8*. Also in: *Indications for Child Analysis and Other Papers*. London: Hogarth Press, 1969.

Freud, A. (1957). The contribution of direct child observation to psychoanalysis. In: *The Writings of Anna Freud, Vol. 5*   . New York: International Universities Press, 1969.

Freud, S. (1905d). *Three Essays on the Theory of Sexuality. S.E., 7*.

Freud, S. (1910d). The future prospects of psycho-analytic therapy. *S.E., 11*.

Freud, S. (1910i). The psycho-analytic view of psychogenic disturbance of vision. *S.E., 11*.

Freud, S. (1911b). Formulations on the two principles of mental functioning. *S.E., 12*.

Freud, S. (1912e). Recommendations to physicians practising psychoanalysis. *S.E., 12*.

Freud, S. (1915a). Observations on transference-love. *S.E., 12*.

Freud, S. (1916–17). *Introductory Lectures on Psycho-Analysis. S.E., 15–16*.

Freud, S. (1920g). *Beyond the Pleasure Principle. S.E., 18*.

Freud, S. (1923a [1922]). Two encyclopeadia articles. *S.E., 18*.

Freud, S. (1923b). *The Ego and the Id. S.E., 19*.

Galison, P., & Stump, D. J. (Eds.) (1996).*The Disunity of Science: Boundaries, Contexts and Powers*. Stanford, CA: Stanford University Press.

Gardziel, A. (2002). A history of the early years of Esther Bick. *International Journal of Infant Observation and Its Applications, 5* (2).

Geertz, C. (1973). *The Interpretation of Cultures*. New York: Basic Books.

Gell-Mann, M. (1994). *The Quark and the Jaguar: Adventures in the Simple and the Complex*. London: Abacus.

Gitelson, M. (1949). The emotional position of the analyst in the psycho-analytic situation. *International Journal of Psycho-Analysis, 33*.

Gleick, J. (1998). *Chaos and the Science of the Unpredictable* . London: Vintage.

Goffman, I. (1961). *Asylums*. London: Penguin, 1968.

Grotstein, J. (1981). Wilfred R. Bion: the man, the psychoanalyst, the mystic. A perspective on his life and work. In: *Do I Dare Disturb the Universe? A Memorial to Wilfred R. Bion.* Beverly Hills, CA: Caesura Press.

Grunbaum, A. (1984). *The Foundations of Psychoanalysis: A Philosophical Critique.* Los Angeles: University of California Press.

Grunbaum, A. (1993). *Validation in the Clinical Theory of Psychoanalysis.* Madison, CT: International Universities Press.

Haag, G. (1991). Some reflections on body ego development through psychotherapeutic work with an infant. In: R. Szur & S. Miller (Eds.), *Extending Horizons.* London: Karnac.

Haag, G. (2000). In the footsteps of Frances Tustin: further reflections on the construction of the body ego. *International Journal of Infant Observation and Its Applications, 3:* 7–22.

Harris, M. (1975). *Thinking about Infants and Young Children.* Strathtay: Clunie Press.

Harris, M. (1982). Growing pains in psychoanalysis inspired by the work of Melanie Klein. *Journal of Child Psychotherapy , 8* (2): 165–184.

Harris, M. (1983). Esther Bick (1901–1983).   *Journal of Child Psychotherapy, 9.*

Healy, K. (1998). Clinical audit and conflict. In: R. Davenhill & M. Patrick (Eds.), *Rethinking Clinical Audit.* London: Routledge.

Hindle, D., & Easton, J. (1999). The use of observation of supervised contact in child care cases. *The International Journal of Infant Observation and Its Applications, 2* (2).

Hinshelwood, R. D. (1999). The difficult patient: the role of "scientific" psychiatry in understanding patients with chronic schizophrenia or severe personality disorder. *British Journal of Psychiatry, 174* : 187–190.

Hinshelwood, R. D., & Skogstad, W. (2000). *Observing Organisations .* London: Routledge.

Hollway, W., & Jefferson, T. (2000). *Doing Qualitative Research Differently: Free Association, Narrative and the Interview Method .* London: Sage.

Hopkins, J. (1996). The dangers and deprivations of too-good mothering. *Journal of Child Psychotherapy, 23* (2): 407–422.

Houzel, D. (2001a). The bisexuality of the psychic envelope. In J.

Edwards (Ed.), *Being Alive: Building on the Work of Anne Alvarez*. London & New York: Brunner-Routledge.

Houzel, D. (2001b). "Splitting of Psychic Bisexuality in Autistic Children." Paper read at the European Federation for Psychoanalytic Psychotherapy Conference on Psychosis and Childhood and Adolescence, Caen, 30 September.

Jaques, E. (1953). On the dynamics of social structure.*Human Relations*, 6: 10–23.

Jaques, E. (1955). The social system as a defence against anxiety. In: M. Klein, P. Heimann, and R. Money-Kyrle (Eds.), *New Directions in Psychoanalysis*. London: Tavistock.

Joseph, B. (1975). The patient who is difficult to reach. In P. L. Giovacchini (Ed.), *Tactics and Techniques in Psychoanalytic Therapy, Vol. 2: Countertransference*. New York: Jason Aronson. Also in E. B. Spillius (Ed.), *Melanie Klein Today, Vol. 2: Mainly Practice*. London: Routledge, 1988; E. B. Spillius & M. Feldman (Eds.),*Psychic Equilibrium and Psychic Change: Selected Papers of Betty Joseph*. London & New York: Tavistock/Routledge.

Joseph, B. (1989). *Psychic Equilibrium and Psychic Change*. London: Routledge.

Joseph, B. (1994). "Where there is no vision." From sexualisation to sexuality. *Bulletin of the British Psychoanalytical Society, 30* (10).

Kaës, R., & Anzieu, D. (Eds.) (1993). *Les Contenants de Pensée*. Paris: Dunod.

Kauffman, S. (1995). *At Home in the Universe*. London: Viking.

Keats, J. (1817). Letter to George and Tom Keats, 21 (or 27) December. In: *Letters of John Keats*, ed. R. Gittings. Oxford: Oxford University Press, 1987.

Keats, J. (1819). Letter to George and Georgiana, 19 March. In:*Letters of John Keats*, ed. R. Gittings. Oxford: Oxford University Press, 1987.

Klein, M. (1923). Early analysis. In: *Love, Guilt and Reparation and Other Works. The Writings of Melanie Klein, Vol. 1*. London: Hogarth Press, 1975.

Klein, M. (1927). Symposium on child analysis. In: *Love, Guilt and Reparation and Other Works. The Writings of Melanie Klein, Vol. 1* London: Hogarth Press, 1975.

Klein, M. (1932). *The Psycho-Analysis of Children*. London: Hogarth Press.

Klein, M. (1940). Mourning and its relation to manic-depressive states. In: *Love, Guilt and Reparation and Other Works. The Writings of Melanie Klein, Vol. 1*. London, Hogarth Press, 1975.

Klein, M. (1946). Notes on some schizoid mechanisms. In: *Envy and Gratitude and Other Works. The Writings of Melanie Klein, Vol. 3*. London: Hogarth Press, 1975.

Klein, S. (1980). Autistic phenomena in neurotic patients. *International Journal of Psycho-Analysis, 61*: 395–402. Also in J. S. Grotstein (Ed.), *Do I Dare Disturb the Universe?* Beverly Hills, CA: Caesura Press, 1981.

Knorr-Cetina, K. (1999). *Epistemic Cultures: How the Sciences Make Knowledge*. Cambridge, MA: Harvard University Press.

Kolvin, I., Macmillan, A., Nicol, A. R., & Wrate, R. M. (1988). Psychotherapy is effective. *Journal of the Royal Society of Medicine , 81* (5): 261–266.

Kuhn, T. S. (1962). *The Structure of Scientific Revolutions*. Chicago, IL: Chicago University Press.

Laplanche, J., & Pontalis, B. (1973).   *The Language of Psychoanalysis*. London: Karnac, 1988.

Lask, B., Britten, C., Kroll, L., Magagna, J., & Tranter, M. (1991). Pervasive refusal in children. *Archives of Disease in Childhood, 66* : 866–869.

Lecourt, E. (1990). The musical envelope. In: D. Anzieu (Ed.),   *Psychic Envelopes*. London: Karnac.

Likierman, M. (1989). The clinical significance of aesthetic experience. *International Review of Psycho-Analysis, 16* (2).

Magagna, J. (1986). Della pelle della madre. In: M. Pontecorvo   (Ed.), *Esperienze di psicoterapia infantile: Il modello Tavistock*. Rome: Psycho di Martinelli & Firenze.

Magagna, J., & Dubinsky, H. (1983). Remembering Mrs Bick remembering Mrs Klein. *Tavistock Gazette, 10*.

Main, M., & Hesse, E. (1990). Parents' unresolved traumatic experiences are related to infant disorganised attachment status: is frightened and/or frightening parental behaviour the linking mechanism? In: M Greenbg, D. Cicchetti, & E. M. Cummings (Eds.), *Attachment in the Pre-School Years: Theory, Research and Intervention* (pp. 161–182). Chicago, IL: Chicago University Press.

Main, M., & Solomon, J. (1986). Discovery of an insecure/disorganised/disoriented attachment pattern. In: T. B. Brazelton & M. W.

Yogman (Ed.), *Affective Development in Infancy* (pp. 95–125). Norwood, NJ: Ablex.

Malinowski, B. (1923). Psychoanalysis and anthropology. *Nature, 112*: 650–651.

Mandelbrot, B. B. (1977). *The Fractal Geometry of Nature* (rev. ed.). New York: W. H. Freeman, 1983.

McDougall, J. (1985). Psychosomatic states, anxiety neurosis and hysteria. In: *Theaters of the Mind: Illusion and Truth on the Psychoanalytic Stage.* New York: Basic Books.

Meltzer, D. (1967). *The Psycho-Analytical Process.* London: Heinemann.

Meltzer, D. (1974). Adhesive identification. In: *Sincerity and Other Works: The Collected Papers of Donald Meltzer*, ed. A. Hahn. London: Karnac, 1994.

Meltzer, D. (1975). *Explorations in Autism.* Strathtay: Clunie Press.

Meltzer, D. (1986a). Discussion of Esther Bick's Paper "Further Consideration of the Function of the Skin in Early Object Relations". *British Journal of Psychotherapy, 2* (4): 300–301.

Meltzer, D. (1986b). *Studies in Extended Metapsychology.* Strathtay: Clunie Press.

Meltzer, D., & Harris Williams, M. (1988). *The Apprehension of Beauty: The Role of Aesthetic Conflict in Development, Art and Violence* Strathtay: Clunie Press.

Meltzer, D. (1992). *The Claustrum: An Investigation of Claustrophobic Phenomena.* Strathtay: Clunie Press.

Menzies, I. (1959). A case study in the functioning of the social system as a defence against anxiety. *Human Relations, 113* : 95–121. Reprinted in: I. Menzies Lyth, *Containing Anxiety in Institutions.* London: Free Association Books, 1988.

Miller, L., Rustin, M. E., Rustin, M. J., & Shuttleworth, J. (Eds.) (1989). *Closely Observed Infants.* London: Duckworth.

Miller, M. L. (1999). Chaos, complexity and psychoanalysis. *Psychoanalytic Psychology, 16* (3).

Moran, M. H. (1991). Chaos theory and psychoanalysis: the fluidistic nature of the mind. *International Review of Psycho-Analysis, 18* (2): 211–221.

Obholzer, A., & Roberts, V. (1994). *The Unconscious at Work* . London: Routledge.

OFSTED (1996). *The Education of Travellers' Children.* London: OFSTED Publications Centre.

Okley, J. (1983). *The Traveller-Gypsies*. Cambridge: Cambridge University Press.

O'Shaughnessy, E. (1964). The absent object. *Journal of Child Psychotherapy, 1*: 34–43.

O'Shaughnessy, E. (1994). What is a clinical fact?' *International Journal of Psycho-Analysis, 75*: 939–947.

Pines, D. (1980). Skin communication: early skin disorders and their effect on transference and countertransference. *International Journal of Psycho-Analysis, 61*: 315–322. Reprinted in: *A Woman's Unconscious Use of Her Body*. London: Virago Press, 1993.

Poincaré, H. (1908). *Science and Method*. New York: Dover, 1952.

Prigogine, I. (1996). *The End of Certainty*. New York: Free Press.

Prigogine, I., & Stengers, I. (1984). *Order Out of Chaos*. New York: Bantam.

Quinodoz, J.-M. (1997). Transitions in psychic structures in the light of deterministic chaos theory. *International Journal of Psycho-Analysis, 78* (4): 699–718.

Reid, S. (1997). The generation of psychoanalytic knowledge: sociological and clinical perspectives, Part 2. Projective identification: the other side of the equation. *British Journal of Psychotherapy , 13* (4): 542–554.

Resnik, S. (1995). *Mental Space*. London: Karnac.

Rey, H. (1994). *Universals in Psychoanalysis*. London: Free Association Books.

Rhode, M. (1997a). Going to pieces: autistic and schizoid solutions. In: M. Rustin, M. Rhode, A. Dubinsky, & H. Dubinsky (Eds.),*Psychotic States in Children*. London: Duckworth/Tavistock Clinic Series.

Rhode, M. (1997b). Psychosomatic integrations: eye and mouth in infant observation. In: S. Reid (Ed.), *Developments in Infant Observation: The Tavistock Model*. London & New York: Routledge.

Rhode, M. (2000). On using an alphabet: recombining separable components. In J. Symington (Ed.), *Imprisoned Pain and Its Transformation: A Festschrift for H. Sydney Klein*. London: Karnac.

Robinson, S. (2002). What gets measured, gets delivered? *Psychoanalytic Psychotherapy, 16* (1): 37–57.

Ruelle, D. (1991). *Chance and Chaos*. Harmondsworth: Penguin.

Rustin, M. E. (2001). The therapist with her back against the wall. *Journal of Child Psychotherapy, 27*: 273–284.

Rustin, M. J. (1989). Observing infants: reflections on methods. In: L.

Miller, M. E. Rustin, M. J. Rustin, & J. Shuttleworth (Eds.),   *Closely Observed Infants*. London: Duckworth.

Rustin, M. J. (1991a).   *The Good Society and the Inner World.*   London: Verso.

Rustin, M. J. (1991b). Psychoanalysis, philosophical realism, and the new sociology of science. In: *The Good Society and the Inner World.* London: Verso.

Rustin, M. J. (1991c). Psychoanalysis and aesthetic experience. In: *The Good Society and the Inner World.* London: Verso.

Rustin, M. J. (1997). What do we see in the nursery?   *International Journal of Infant Observation,*   1 (1). Reprinted in: *Reason and Unreason: Psychoanalysis, Science and Politics*   . London: Continuum, 2001.

Rustin, M. J. (2001a).   *Reason and Unreason: Psychoanalysis, Science and Politics.* London: Continuum.

Rustin, M. J. (2001b). Research, evidence and psychotherapy. In: C. Mace, S. Moorey, & B. Roberts (Eds.),   *Evidence in the Balance: A Critical Guide for Practitioners*   . Hove: Brunner-Routledge. Reprinted in: *Reason and Unreason: Psychoanalysis, Science and Politics.* London: Continuum, 2001.

Salzberger-Wittenberg, I. (1983).   *The Emotional Experience of Learning and Teaching.* London: Routledge & Kegan Paul.

Scheff, T. (1997).   *Emotions, the Social Bond and Human Reality: Part/ Whole Analysis.* Cambridge: Cambridge University Press.

Segal, H. (1957). Notes on symbol formation. In: E. B. Spillius (Ed.), *Melanie Klein Today: Vol. 1.* London: Routledge, 1988.

Sorensen, P. B. (2000). Observations of transition facilitating behaviour—developmental and theoretical implications.   *International Journal of Infant Observation,* 3 (2).

Spillius, E. B. (1988). *Melanie Klein Today, Vol. 1: Mainly Theory; Vol. 2: Mainly Practice.* London: Routledge.

Steiner, J. (1993). *Psychic Retreats.* London: Routledge.

Stern, D. (1983). The early development of schemas of Self, Other and Self with Other. In: J. D. Lichtenberg & S. Kaplan (Eds.), *Reflections on Self Psychology.* London: Analytic Press.

Stewart, I. (1990). *Does God Play Dice? The New Mathematics of Chaos* London: Penguin.

Strachey, J. (1934). The nature of the therapeutic action of psychoanalysis. *International Journal of Psycho-Analysis,* 15: 127–159.

Symington, J. (1985). The survival function of primitive omnipotence. *International Journal of Psycho-Analysis, 66*: 481–487.

Taylor, M. C. (2001). *The Moment of Complexity: Emerging Network Culture*. Chicago, IL: Chicago University Press.

Thom, R. (1975). *Structural Stability and Morphogenesis: An Outline of a General Theory of Models*. Reading: Benjamin.

Thrift, N. (1999). The place of complexity. *Theory, Culture and Society, 3*: 31–69.

Trevarthen, C. (1998). The concept and foundations of infant intersubjectivity. In: S. Braten (Ed.), *Intersubjective Communication and Emotion in Early Ontogeny*. Cambridge: Cambridge University Press.

Trist, E. (1950). Culture as a psychosocial process. In E. Trist & H. Murray (Eds.), *The Social Engagement of Social Science*. London: Free Association Books, 1990.

Trist, E., & Murray, H. (Eds.) (1990). *The Social Engagement of Social Science*. London: Free Association Books.

Trowell, J. (1999). Assessments and court work: the place of observation. *International Journal of Infant Observation and Its Applications, 2* (2).

Trowell, J., & Miles, G. (1991). The place of an introduction to young child observation in social work training. In: *The Teaching of Child Care in the Diploma of Social Work: Guidance Notes for Programme Planners* (pp. 130–139). London: CCETSW.

Trowell, J., & Rustin, M. (1991). Developing the internal observer in professionals in training. *Infant Mental Health Journal, 12*: 233–245.

Tustin, F. (1972). *Autism and Childhood Psychosis*. London: Hogarth Press. Reprinted London: Karnac, 1995.

Tustin, F. (1981a). *Autistic States in Children* (revised edition). London: Routledge, 1992.

Tustin, F. (1981b). Psychological birth and psychological catastrophe. In: *Autistic States in Children* (revised edition). London: Routledge, 1992. Also in J. S. Grotstein (Ed.), *Do I Dare Disturb the Universe?* Beverly Hills, CA: Caesura Press, 1981.

Tustin, F. (1986). *Autistic Barriers in Neurotic Patients*. London: Karnac.

Tustin, F. (1990). *The Protective Shell in Children and Adults*. London: Karnac.

Waldrop, M. M. (1992). *Complexity: The Emerging Science at the Edge of Order and Chaos*. New York: Simon & Schuster.

Wengraf, T. (2001). Uncovering the general from within the particular: from contingencies to typologies in the understanding of cases. In: P. M. Chamberlayne, J. Bornat, & T. Wengraf (Eds.),   *The Turn to Biographical Methods in Social Science.* London: Taylor & Francis/ Routledge.

Will, D. (1980). Psychoanalysis as a human science.   *British Journal of Medical Psychology, 53*: 201–211.

Will, D. (1986). Psychoanalysis and the new philosophy of science. *International Review of Psychoanalysis, 13*: 163–173.

Williams, G. (1997a). *Internal Landscapes and Foreign Bodies: Eating Disorders and Other Pathologies.* London: Duckworth/Tavistock Clinic Series.

Williams, G. (1997b). On the process of internalisation. In: *Internal Landscapes and Foreign Bodies: Eating Disorders and Other Pathologies.* London: Duckworth/Tavistock Clinic Series.

Willoughby, R. (2001). The petrified self: Esther Bick and her membership paper. *British Journal of Psychotherapy, 18* (1).

Winnicott, D. W. (1949). Birth memories, birth trauma, and anxiety. In: *Through Paediatrics to Psycho-Analysis.* London: Tavistock, 1958. Reprinted London: Karnac, 1992.

Winnicott, D. W. (1951). Transitional objects and transitional phenomena. In: *Through Paediatrics to Psycho-Analysis,* London: Hogarth Press, 1958. Reprinted London: Karnac, 1992. Also in: *Playing and Reality.* London & New York: Routledge/Tavistock Publications, 1971.

Winnicott, D. W. (1960). The thory of the parent–infant relationship. In: *The Maturational Processes and the Facilitating Environment.* London: Hogarth Press, 1965. Reprinted London: Karnac, 1990.

Winnicott, D. W. (1967). Mirror-role of mother and family in child development. In: *Playing and Reality.* London & New York: Routledge/Tavistock Publications, 1971.

Wittenberg, I. (1975). Primal depression in autism—John. In: D. Meltzer, J. Bremner, S. Hoxter, D. Weddell, & I. Wittenberg, *Explorations in Autism.* Strathtay: Clunie Press.

Woodcock, A., & Davis, M. (1980).   *Catastrophe Theory* . Harmondsworth: Penguin.

Youell, B. (1999). From observation to work with a child . *International Journal of Infant Observation and Its Applications, 2* (2).

Young, E. B. (1996). A psychoanalytic approach to addiction: the formation and use of a precocious paranoid-schizoid-depressive organisation. *Journal of Melanie Klein and Object Relations, 14* 177–195.

Zeeman, C. (1977). *Catastrophe Theory: Selected Papers 1972–1977*. Reading: Benjamin.

INDEX

Printed in the United States
by Baker & Taylor Publisher Services